Allergies and their Management

Allergies and their Management

Ronald S. Walls
MBChB D Phil (Oxon) FCP(SA) FRACP FRCPA

Associate Professor of Medicine
University of Sydney
and
Director of Clinical Immunology and Allergy
Concord Repatriation General Hospital

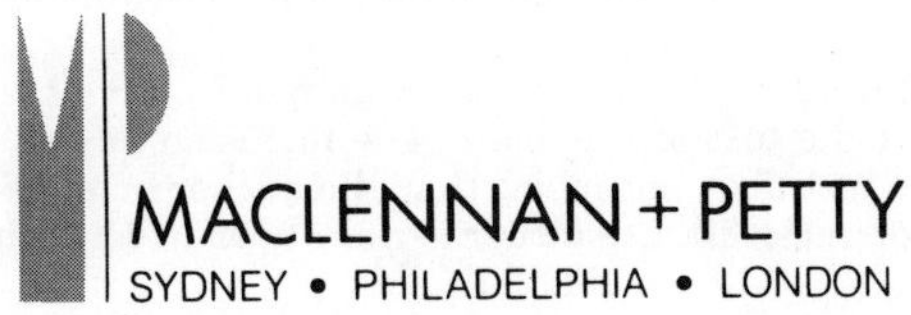

First published 1997

MacLennan & Petty Pty Limited
4/809 Botany Road, Rosebery, Sydney NSW 2018 Australia

National Library of Australia
Cataloguing-in-Publication data:

Allergies and their Management

Bibliography
Includes index

ISBN 0 86433 115 0

Printed and bound in Australia

Contents

Part A. Basic Principles of Diagnosis and Management

Part B. Applied Clinical Practice

Part C. Basic Mechanisms in Allergic Diseases

Foreword

In the middle of the 16th century the distinguished Italian physician Gerome Cardan was summonsed all the way from Pavia to Edinburgh to attend the Reverend John Hamilton, Archbishop of St Andrews, who had suffered from sporadic and crippling dyspnoea for 10 years. Having made the diagnosis of asthma, Cardan 'cured' the overweight cleric by diet, regular exercise and sleep, and by prohibiting the use of feathers in his bed. Although this episode is hardly complimentary to the practice of allergy in Great Britain at the time, it does encapsulate the essence of allergic disease by highlighting the need for a correct diagnosis followed by the implementation of simple but effective therapy. During the intervening years between Cardan's visit to Edinburgh and the coining of the term 'allergy' by von Pirquet in 1906, the allergic basis of other conditions like summer catarrh or hay fever and hives was recognised, often by clinicians who suffered from them personally. It is therefore somewhat surprising that a group of common disorders with such a long history still poses a very real challenge to the clinician today.

Professor Ron Walls has taken up the gauntlet and has produced a book which should have wide appeal to those in training, as well as to those in practice. There are several reasons for this: firstly, he has a wealth of practical experience spanning 30 years in conjunction with a sound background in immunological principles; secondly, the book is eminently readable unlike some of the discursive, albeit erudite, texts published previously. By virtue of the format, one does not have to wade through numerous pages to find what one wants, but can select the section of relevance to the particular clinical problem. When a little more time is available, there is plenty of information on and references to underlying mechanisms and the rationale behind various forms of therapy. Thirdly, the author has made a special point of distinguishing between the fact, fiction and surmise which have bedevilled the field of allergic disease for many years. Finally, he has chosen to include some of the more controversial aspects of the practice of allergy, such as multiple chemical sensitivities, chronic fatigue syndrome and behavioural disturbances. This is sensible since patients with these conditions tend to gravitate to practitioners in the field of allergy and it is vital that they be cared for by those with appropriate qualifications.

The book is divided into three main sections. Section 1 encompasses the principles of diagnosis and management, including prevention, diet, drugs and immunotherapy, and makes a very readable package. It is followed by a section dealing with the various clinical entities which bring the patient to the doctor. Their selection is comprehensive, including well recognised conditions such as urticaria, rhinitis and asthma, as well as newer disorders like latex sensitivity which is being seen by medical, paramedical and dental practitioners in almost epidemic proportions. The third and final section provides an outline of the basic mechanisms underlying allergic disease, and their clinical manifestations. The importance of environmental and genetic factors, in addition to IgE, eosinophils and basophils, is given appropriate weight. For those who require more specific details on management issues the appendices offer information on protocols and various support services in Australia.

Professor Walls is to be congratulated on producing a text which is not only readable but contains a wealth of practical as well as basic information on a group of disorders comprising 15% of general practice and presenting many challenges for the specialist physician. On reading this book, any student of medicine, uncertain about his or her future, will be impressed with the diverse opportunities offered by a career in clinical allergy.

Professor Antony Basten
AO, FAA, FTSE, MBBS, D Phil (Oxon), FRACP, FRCPA, FRCP
Director, Centenary Institute of Cancer Medicine and Cell Biology
Professor of Immunology and Head of Department
of Experimental Medicine, University of Sydney

Preface

Allergic diseases are among the most common of all conditions confronting primary care physicians, yet many of these general practitioners have had little or no formal training in this important branch of medical practice. There are a number of reasons for this. Allergies are not commonly encountered in hospital practice, and so medical students have little, if any, experience of them before going into practice. There used to be no formal teaching in allergic diseases at medical schools, but this situation has changed for the better in recent years. It is only in the last year that an academic department of allergy was established at an Australian university. There is also a perception that allergies are trivial disorders, and that modern drugs are so effective in controlling symptoms that there is no need to spend a lot of time investigating them. Adequate clinical assessment is time-consuming as it needs to take into account the influence of environmental factors on the disease. Allergies are diseases of our modern society and there is evidence of an alarming increase in the incidence of these diseases throughout the world. The reasons for this are by no means clear, although there are a number of theories.

The aims of the book are three-fold. Firstly, to provide a practical, readily accessed guide to recognition and clinical management of allergic problems. Secondly, to provide a basic background in the scientific disciplines relevant to allergy, to enable the user to understand the basis of clinical practice. The book has been designed in such a way that this background material does not interfere with its use as a handbook or practical guide. And thirdly, to indicate controversial areas of practice and identify those which have been shown to be ineffective. Algorithms are provided in some chapters, but these are illustrative only and cannot replace clinical judgment in the individual patient.

This book is offered as a guide for medical practitioners not primarily involved in allergy practice, and for residents and students who will surely be confronted by these conditions at some time in their careers. There is a limited amount of detail by necessity, but it is hoped that appetites will be whetted and readers will be moved to consult one of the more detailed texts or review articles from time to time. I hope the book also manages to convey the message that these are fascinating disorders if one looks behind and beyond the symptoms.

I would like to thank many colleagues who have shared their knowledge and enthusiasm, and contributed thereby in no small measure to this book. I would especially like to thank Dr Diana Bass for reading some of the text, and for valuable advice, particularly in relation to aerobiology and pollen distribution. Other colleagues who have provided information on pollen distribution around Australia are Professor D. Czarny and Drs C. Katelaris, G. Solley, J. Weiner and R. Heddle.

Chapter 1

What is allergy? An introduction

Definition

The word 'allergy' has lost its original biological meaning in everyday language and has come to mean a dislike or aversion. Allergy was originally defined as the altered reaction which occurs when an antigen is administered to a subject after an original immunising dose. The immune response to subsequent doses of antigen is qualitatively and quantitatively different from the one following the first dose. Medical usage of the term 'allergy' has become more restricted to immunological reactions mediated by IgE antibodies and which manifest as the allergic diseases such as asthma, hayfever, urticaria, and anaphylaxis. Allergic diseases are all caused by external environmental agents, and therefore tend to affect organs at the interface with the external environment.

'Atopy' is a term first coined by Coca and Cooke in 1923 to refer to the clinical manifestations of allergy. They recognised that there was a hereditary element and that serum factors, termed 'reagins' (which we now know to be IgE), were responsible for these diseases. A group of the population, numbering up to 40%, who have the predilection for producing an IgE mediated response to antigens are now described as being atopic. These people are characterised by the presence of allergic disease, show evidence of IgE production by demonstrating a positive reaction to skin prick tests and have a family history of allergic diseases.

History

Allergic diseases were described well before this century, and may have even changed the course of history. Perhaps the earliest report is that of King Menes of Egypt who was killed by the sting of a 'great wasp' at some time between 3640 and 3300 BC while on a visit to the Western Isles (a possible reference to Britain). Another report from ancient history is that of Britannicus, the son of the Roman Emperor Claudius, so named in honour of his father's successful conquest of Britain. Britannicus was allergic to horses, developed a rash and his eyes swelled to the extent that he could not see where he was going. Accordingly, the honour of riding at the head of the young patricians fell to Nero who was Claudius's adopted son. Nero, of course, has been credited with burning Rome, throwing Christians to the lions, and killing Britannicus. Sir Thomas More gave the next authoritative account of allergy. King Richard III used his allergy to strawberries to good effect in arranging the judicial murder of Lord William Hastings. The king

FIGURE 1.1 **Charles Blackley with a pollen trap on a kite**.

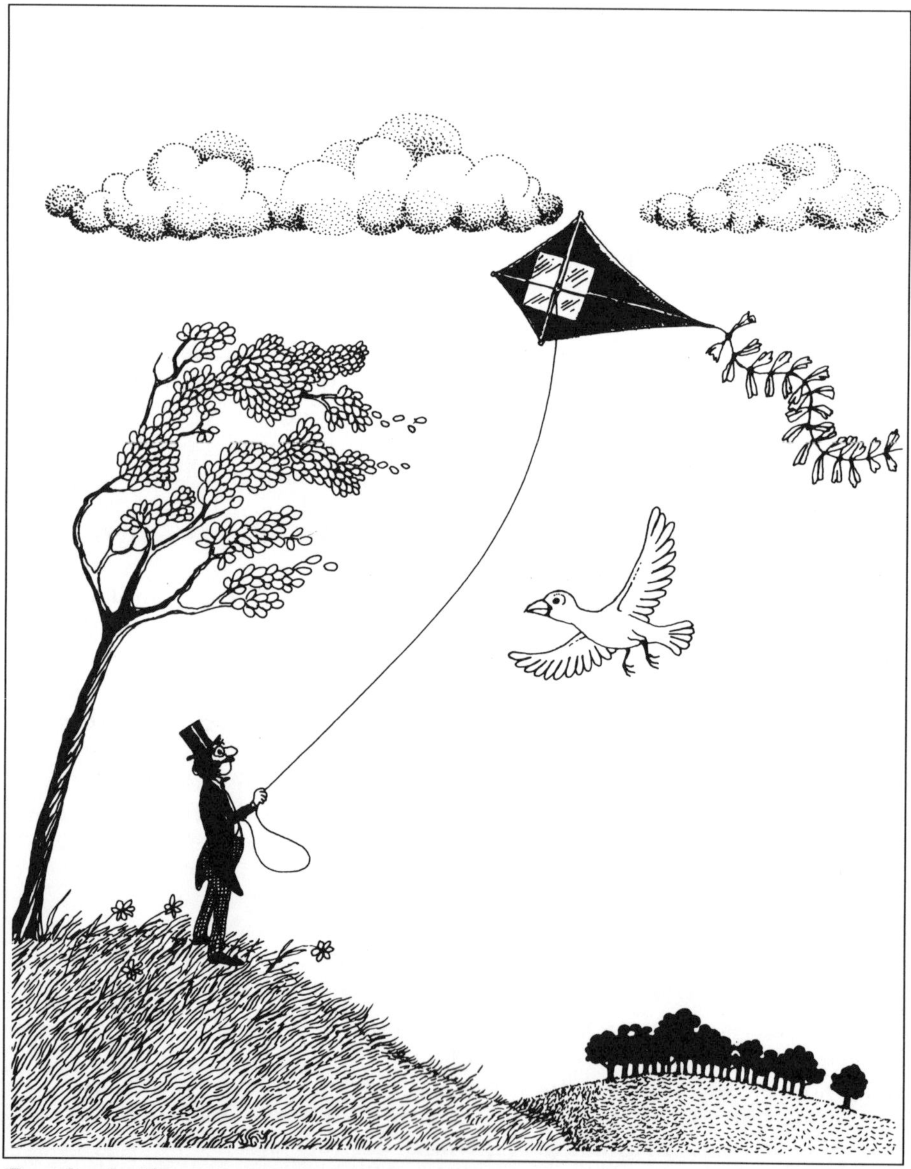

(Reproduced with permission from Avenberg KM, Harper SM, Larsson BL. Footnotes on allergy. Uppsala: Pharmacia AB, 1980).

surreptitiously ate some strawberries just prior to giving an audience to Hastings and promptly developed acute urticaria. He then accused the hapless nobleman of putting a curse on him, an action which demanded the head of Hastings on a plate.

Hayfever was described for the first time in the early part of the 19th century by Bostock, who was himself an asthmatic. The term *'catarrhus aestivus'* was given to this malady, but only 28 cases could be identified in the whole of Britain. Charles Blackley of Manchester, whose name has been immortalised in the world of allergy, made strenuous efforts to prove that pollen was the cause of hayfever. He collected and sniffed them six months after the pollen season, and was able to produce typical hayfever symptoms. He did a skin test by rubbing pollen into a scratch on his arm and elicited a violent reaction like a nettle rash. He was the father of allergy, but also of aerobiology. He covered glass plates with glycerine and sent them up 500 metres into the atmosphere on kites where he was able to collect pollen grains, thereby showing that pollen can be transported in the air.

In 1900 Richet and Portier, two French physicians, described the unexpected death of laboratory animals following the injection of actinotoxin found in the tentacles of the Portuguese man-of-war *(Physalia physalis)*. Instead of the first injection protecting the animals (prophylaxis) as the physicians were expecting, the animals developed increased sensitivity and died soon after the injection. Richet and Portier coined the term 'anaphylaxis' to describe this phenomenon. In 1906 Clemens von Pirquet used the word 'allergy' for the first time to describe the altered reactivity to subsequent exposure to antigens.

During this century a cadre of physicians with a special interest in allergic diseases has developed. These doctors originally came from the ranks of general practice where they came across these diseases in many of their patients. A bank of knowledge was built up over this century from clinical experience, but there was little scientific understanding of the specialty until 1966 when Ishizaka and Ishizaka and Bennich and Johansson described a new immunoglobulin molecule which they termed 'IgE' and which was responsible for mediating the allergic response. Since then there has been a rapid advance in our knowledge of the biology of the allergic response. The biochemistry and synthesis of the mediators of the allergic reaction have been clarified, and an understanding of the role of T cells, cytokines and adhesion molecules has led to an appreciation of the importance of inflammatory processes in the allergic reaction. More recently allergy has been recognised as a specialty in clinical immunology, and the responsibility for training has been assumed by the Royal Australasian College of Physicians.

What are allergists?

The role of the allergy specialist is to determine whether allergic processes are contributing to disease in an individual and to identify the offending allergens. They may need to determine whether environmental agents are contributing to disease by other than IgE mediated mechanisms. They must be able to advise on avoidance techniques and the risks of developing allergic diseases in certain occupations. They need to be able to advise on and select treatment options other than purely pharmacological, and this may include immunotherapy. They may be called upon to advise on public health measures such as the planting of low-pollinating plants.

Allergy specialists need to have knowledge and proficiency in three areas over and above the traditional skills of the clinician. The first is a knowledge of environmental allergens, their behaviour under different conditions, where they are found and effective control measures. Secondly, they need to be familiar with the use of specific diagnostic tests to identify the cause of allergies. These tests are primarily skin prick tests, but challenge or provocation tests are also required at times. The third is the use of specific immune therapy. Effective allergy practice needs access to nursing services highly skilled in allergy management and to the services of dieticians with specific expertise and interest in adverse reactions to foods.

Children constitute a large proportion of the total allergic population. The presentation and natural history of disease in this age group differs from that of adults and their management requires different emphasis from adults. Great care must be taken with dietary investigations as children are particularly vulnerable to inappropriate dietary restriction. It is important that allergists with training in paediatrics be available for this population.

What are allergic diseases?

One outstanding feature of allergic diseases is that they involve organs in contact with the external environment. Allergic diseases are among the most common reasons why patients consult their family doctors. They affect the younger age group predominantly, and therefore have a disproportionately severe socio-economic effect on the community in terms of absenteeism, interference with ability to work, study and lifestyle, and costs of medication.

Allergic diseases seem to be a by-product of modern civilisation. There has been an alarming increase in respiratory allergies in the last 25 years in Western countries, particularly the English-speaking world. Countries such as those of Eastern Europe which have been sheltered from modern technocratic cultures have a much lower rate of allergy, and it will be extremely important to follow the epidemiology of these diseases as the countries develop a Western culture. Populations with heavy worm infestations and many infectious illnesses seem to have a low prevalence of allergic diseases. IgE in evolutionary terms was an important protective mechanism for parasitic disease. It acted as gatekeeper, allowing tissue fluids rich in inflammatory mediators access into sites of infestation.

Does allergy really matter?

Despite the high prevalence of allergic diseases in the community and their undoubted socio-economic impact, allergy remains one of the Cinderella disciplines in medicine. There are a number of reasons for this. There is a misconception that allergies are trivial complaints not worthy of major effort.

However, they cause considerable morbidity in terms of impairment of quality of life and are one of the more common causes of absenteeism in the younger working and studying community. Some allergic conditions such as asthma and anaphylaxis also carry a mortality rate. It has also attracted a larger number of dubious diagnostic and therapeutic practices than most other specialties, and there is a tendency to tar the whole discipline with this brush. Allergic diseases do not often cause hospital admissions and until recently allergy was not taught in the undergraduate curriculum. The result has been that many doctors went out into practice with no knowledge of these common conditions.

The question is sometimes raised as to whether an understanding of allergy really matters in modern times with the availability of highly effective pharmaceutical agents. There is now a better understanding of the important role of allergy in initiating and maintaining the inflammatory process in asthma, allergic rhinitis and other allergic diseases. Modern treatment demands the use of anti-inflammatory drugs to suppress this inflammatory process, predominantly with the use of inhaled corticosteroids. However, if there is persisting exposure to the allergen, the stimulus to inflammation remains and therapy is less effective. Furthermore, there is good evidence that identification and removal of allergen can reverse an inflammatory process and lead to resolution of symptoms. Although the evidence is not yet conclusive, it is becoming more apparent that treatment of allergy in these diseases may alter their natural history, for example by preventing the evolution of asthma from allergic rhinitis. An emphasis on allergic mechanisms also draws attention to the multisystem nature of these diseases and the need to treat all aspects of the disease in a given patient.

What of the future?

We can expect a number of important advances in the next ten years. We are starting to understand the importance of the internal environment in homes which predisposes to the accumulation of allergens such as dust mite. Knowledge is accumulating about construction methods and domestic habits which limit the growth of mites and reduce the amount of moulds and other aeroallergens. The same applies to the outside environment. We understand that native flora are in general poor pollinators and hence it may be possible to substitute these for the more prolific imported varieties, thereby influencing pollen counts in a localised environment.

At a therapeutic level antagonists of mediators other than histamine are being developed and trialled, some of which may prove to have valuable anti-inflammatory properties. Antihistamines themselves are highly effective drugs, but further developments are occurring to ensure that they are truly non-sedating and also lack any cardiotoxicity, and others are now available which can be used topically. Second generation agents have anti-allergy properties other than classical H1 receptor blockade, for example on adhesion molecule presentation. The therapeutic significance of these properties still needs to be determined.

Of more fundamental interest is the work on purifying and sequencing allergens which is leading to the production of peptides. These agents can be used to divert the immune response from IgE production to IgG production. They have a high degree of specificity and so it is extremely important to identify the allergens positively. They have the real potential of abolishing the allergic response to certain allergens and of altering the course of disease.

Further reading

Royal College of Physicians and Royal College of Pathologists. Good allergy practice—standards of care for providers and purchasers of allergy services within the National Health Service. *Clin exp Allergy* 1995; 25: 586–95.

Simons FER (ed). Ancestors of allergy. New York: Global Medical Communications, 1994.

PART A

Basic Principles of Diagnosis and Management

Chapter 2

Approach to diagnosis in allergic diseases

Introduction

Allergic diseases result from interactions with allergens and hence most of these diseases affect organs at the interface with the environment, the nose and upper airways, lungs, eyes, skin and gastro-intestinal system. The object of diagnosis is to identify the pathology causing the patient's symptoms. Allergy practice has an additional responsibility to determine whether environmental factors have contributed to the disease and what these factors are.

Three basic questions need to be answered when one sees an allergy patient:

1. What is the diagnosis, eg asthma, urticaria, rhinitis?
2. Is it likely to be caused by an allergic reaction?
3. What is the offending allergen?

Clinical investigation

History

History taking is the most powerful tool in any diagnostic process, but even more so in allergic diseases. Special knowledge is required, for example the likely allergens in a particular area and their biological behaviour under certain conditions. The history should be directed to three purposes:

1. To establish the diagnosis of the clinical condition. Diagnostic features of particular syndromes are covered in individual chapters but certain general principles can be stated. Allergic diseases tend to involve many organ systems, for example allergic rhinitis or eczema in addition to bronchial asthma, and they tend to fluctuate in severity and to remit. For this reason there may be few physical signs at the time of diagnosis despite a history of major disability at other times.

2. To identify the presence of atopy. Although allergic diseases can start at any age, they tend to affect younger age groups. Features suggestive of atopy are early onset of disease, infantile eczema which usually indicates

TABLE 2.1 **Questions to identify potential allergens**

- Can the patient identify particular precipitants?
- Are symptoms seasonal or perennial. If seasonal, which months are the worst?
- Relation to particular locality, e.g. near a particular tree, a particular house or garden
- Effect of moving, e.g. recent holidays in dry inland environments for temperate coastal dwellers, dusty weekender houses or stored sleeping bags
- Time of day. Symptoms from house dust mite are typically worse during the night and in the early morning hours; many plants pollenate in the early hours of the morning
- Time of week
- Weather conditions
- Related to activities, e.g. domestic chores, horse riding
- Pets

Details of house—construction, state of repair, e.g. gutters, damp patches, recent renovations, ventilation, carpeting, maintenance, cleaning, clutter in bedroom, bedding.

a high degree of atopy and often more severe disease, a family history of allergic diseases, and multiple organ involvement.

3. To identify the offending allergen. It is a popular misconception that this is the function of skin tests and RASTs. These procedures determine whether sensitisation has taken place to particular allergens, but not necessarily clinically relevant allergy. The history is the most important tool for this purpose.

Allergens are not the only precipitants of individual episodes of illness even when the disease is primarily allergic in origin. For example, exercise, changes in temperature or irritants can induce symptoms in dust mite allergic individuals because of end-organ hyperresponsiveness.

Physical examination

There may be no abnormal physical signs at the time of presentation. The facial appearance is often characteristic of allergic disease, especially in children. Longstanding and severe nasal obstruction in young children with persistent mouth breathing can result in significant structural changes to the face. The face becomes elongated and this can have detrimental effects on development of bite and later orthodontic problems. In acute sinusitis there is often redness over the malar area and tenderness to pressure. Chronicity of eczema is usually apparent from the thickening (lichenification) of skin. Always examine the flexural areas of arms and legs and behind the neck. In asthma there may be no abnormal physical signs at the time of diagnosis. Auscultation is unreliable in determining the presence of bronchospasm, and reliance should not be put on the presence or absence of wheezing or rhonchi. The nose should always be examined, including in asthmatics who do not complain of nasal symptoms. The ears may show thickening of the tympanic membrane due to previous infection, or fluid in the middle ear due to inadequate drainage through the Eustacean tube.

Physiological measurements

Spirometry is the most commonly performed physiological measurement but suffers the same limitations as physical examination, in that it may be normal at the time of measurement given the remitting nature of many allergic conditions. Ongoing measurements over a period of time may be more helpful to establish a pattern rather than an isolated reading. Peak expiratory flow rates (PEFR) are easily performed with simple and cheap equipment, and give a valid indication of obstruction and reversibility with inhaled β-2 agonists. They can form the basis of self-monitoring by patients and have become a recognised part of the asthma management plan.

Skin prick tests

Skin prick testing (SPT) is an integral part of the assessment of any allergic patient. It is a much maligned procedure, mainly because its purpose and the information it provides is misunderstood. It demonstrates the presence of cell-bound IgE antibody specific to allergens used in the test. This implies previous exposure and sensitisation, but it does not equate with the production of allergic symptoms by the allergen. When properly conducted skin prick tests are highly sensitive and specific, and they are the gold-standard investigation for the demonstration of specific IgE. RASTs provide similar information from a blood test.

The principle of the skin prick test is to introduce a minute amount of

FIGURE 2.1 **Skin prick testing.**

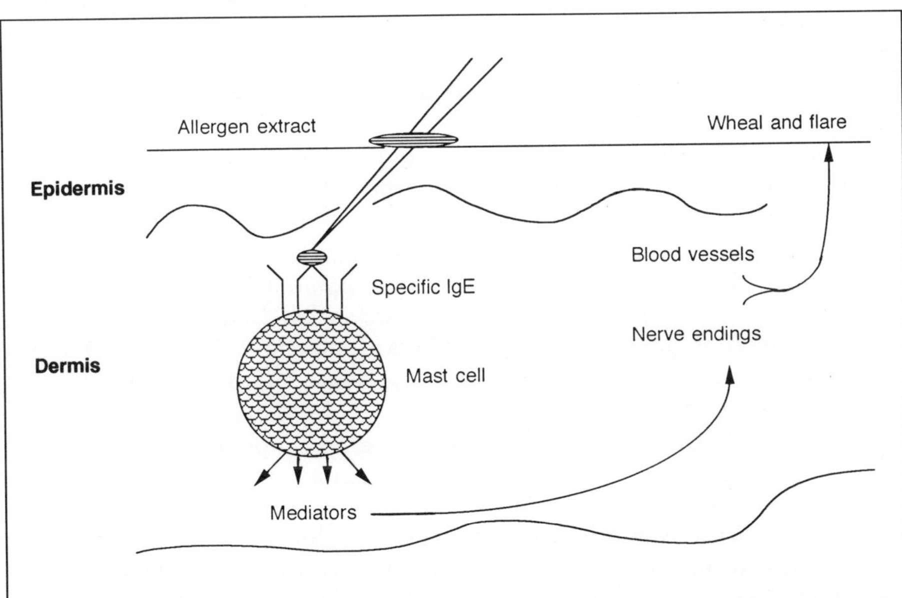

allergen through the epidermis where it combines with specific IgE on the surface of mast cells (Figure 2.1), leading to release of mediators which result in a wheal and flare reaction. Skin test results correlate well with sensitisation in the respiratory tract and elsewhere in the body. Skin test reactivity reaches a peak in the third decade and falls off rapidly after the age of 50 years.

Skin prick tests provide valuable information. They identify the presence of atopy which suggests that allergy may be responsible for the symptoms. They provide support for the historical evidence that a specific allergen is the cause of the patient's symptoms. This is particularly valuable when pollen seasons are erratic, vary from year to year or are prolonged. They may also draw attention to allergens overlooked in the history.

Indications

1. *Asthma.* Every asthmatic deserves an allergy assessment at least once during their illness, and preferably as soon as possible after initial presentation. This may need to be repeated if the clinical picture changes.

2. *Rhinitis.* Identifying that a patient is allergic becomes important where obstruction is the predominant symptom as sometimes occurs with house dust mite allergy, and the paucity of sneezing and rhinorrhoea may mislead one into considering that the patient is non-atopic. The opposite also occurs where particularly watery rhinorrhoea may occur in non-allergic rhinitis, and absence of responses on skin prick testing can be helpful.

3. *Urticaria, angioedema and anaphylaxis.* Skin prick tests help to establish the cause of acute reactions but tend to be negative in chronic urticaria which is a non-atopic disease.

4. *Food allergy.* Skin tests identify specific IgE antibodies which are responsible for acute allergic reactions to foods. Positive results indicating food allergy are more likely to be found in children than adults. Skin tests are of no value for demonstrating food intolerance which is not due to IgE mediated mechanisms.

5. *Atopic eczema.* Skin tests are frequently positive to many allergens as an indication of the atopic state. However, they can also be useful in identifying specific precipitants.

6. *Insect allergy.* Confirmation of an IgE mediated reaction to the venom is always required if immunotherapy is contemplated for a serious reaction. Skin prick tests with the pure venom are reliable but potentially more dangerous than prick testing with inhalant allergens. They should not be undertaken unless the practitioner is experienced in their use and has full resuscitation procedures available.

7. *Drug allergy.* There are few situations where skin prick testing is useful. One problem is the absence of reagents which have been shown to predict accurately the likelihood of future allergic reactions. Another is the fact that most drug reactions are not mediated by IgE mechanisms, including some which appear to have the characteristics of anaphylaxis such as radiographic contrast media. In penicillin allergy, skin tests have been

shown to be reliable predictors of a future severe reaction provided that the appropriate reagents are used.

Procedure

The forearm is the usual site but tests can be performed on the back. The area should be clean but should not be scrubbed, washed or wiped with spirits or antiseptic since these manoeuvres may render the test difficult to interpret. Sensitivity varies with the site selected. Large reactions can reflexly cause positive reactions in adjacent sites, so sufficient space must be left between applications.

Drops of glycerinated allergen extract are placed on the skin and a prick is made through the drop with a blood lancet or a special lancet designed to enter a depth of no more than 1 mm. The volume introduced is 0.006 ml, so great care must be exercised to avoid any carryover from adjacent solutions. Ideally a fresh lancet should be used for each allergen. There should be no bleeding—the presence of blood indicates that the injection was too deep. Excess fluid is dabbed off after 1 minute. The patient often starts experiencing a stinging sensation almost immediately, and within minutes a wheal develops with surrounding erythema (flare). Reactions are maximal at 10 to 15 minutes. A subsequent reaction sometimes develops after about four hours in sensitive subjects due to the late allergic reaction. Histamine acid phosphate 1/1,000 and the glycerosaline vehicle must always be included as positive and negative controls respectively. If histamine is not available a solution of codeine may be used as positive control.

The responses are recorded at 10 minutes for histamine and 15 minutes for allergens. The size of the wheal is recorded in two diameters at right angles to one another, and the mean recorded, or the reaction can be traced with a ballpoint pen and the imprint transferred to paper to provide a permanent record.

Interpretation. A wheal equal to or greater than 3 mm is taken to indicate a positive reaction, provided that there is no reactivity to the negative glycerosaline control. Other criteria sometimes adopted to indicate a positive reaction are a wheal diameter of 2 mm or greater, or a wheal diameter greater than that produced by histamine.

Allergens are selected on the basis of the clinical history and are determined by their prevalence in the area from which the patient comes. Knowledge of the aerobiology in different parts of the country and under different circumstances are essential to allow a meaningful choice of allergens. To identify the presence of atopy it is sufficient to use *Dermatophagoides pteronyssinus,* rye grass pollen, cat and alternaria. It is sometimes necessary to determine whether there is reactivity to allergens for which extracts are not available. The allergen can be extracted with Coca's solution (buffered phenol saline) or the unprocessed material can be placed on the skin and a prick made through it. Under these circumstances a test should also be performed on another person to ensure that any reaction is not due to nonspecific irritation. This procedure should not be carried out with toxic or dangerous substances or where a severe or anaphylactic reaction has occurred, and is best left to specialist allergy practice.

TABLE 2.2 **Drugs which affect reactions to allergens on skin prick testing**

1. *Inhibition of reaction* Antihistamines Antidepressants (especially doxepin) Benzodiazepines Phenothiazines Theophylline β-2 agonists (possibly)	2. *No effect on reaction* Corticosteroids Sodium cromoglycate 3. *Enhancement of reaction* Propranolol β-blockers

Precautions. The risk of an anaphylactic reaction to skin prick testing is very small with inhalant allergens. Nevertheless, it is essential that adrenaline and resuscitative equipment is readily to hand, and that the practitioner is fully conversant with treatment of acute allergic reactions. The likelihood of a reaction to bee or wasp venom or to latex extracts is much greater and it is wise to restrict these tests to specialists or hospital clinics.

Certain drugs interfere with Type 1 reactions, and this is usually indicated by the absence of a reaction to the histamine positive control. Antihistamines should be ceased at least 48 hours before performing skin prick tests, except in the case of astemizole which has a half-life of 21 days, and which after some weeks of therapy can inhibit skin reactivity for 6 weeks. Corticosteroids do not inhibit the Type 1 allergic reaction and do not need to be ceased.

Other techniques for epicutaneous testing, including scratch testing, are no longer performed since skin prick testing is less traumatic and more reproducible and reliable.

With few exceptions, intradermal injection of allergen is not usually performed in allergy assessment. It is used in tailoring the initial dose of immunotherapy in bee sting allergy, and is used for investigating drug allergy. In other situations intradermal tests are too sensitive and have an unacceptable rate of false positive reactions. They do not correlate with clinical manifestations of allergy or with provocation testing. They are also more dangerous than skin prick testing and should not be performed.

Elimination procedures

This process is applied most frequently in the investigation of adverse reactions to foods. However, the same principle can be applied to determine whether improvement occurs when other allergens such as drugs, house dust mite or moulds are exluded from the environment.

Provocation testing

Suspected precipitants can be administered, ideally in a double-blind fashion to determine whether the symptoms can be reproduced. This procedure often follows on from a process of elimination. It is applied most frequently in investigating food reactions (see Chapter 17). It can also be applied in difficult cases of respiratory allergy where it is important to establish whether exposure to an allergen can reproduce the patient's symptoms. In provocation testing the allergen is applied to the target organ under controlled conditions and the reaction observed. The risks with this procedure are greater than with skin prick testing and it should only be undertaken by clinics and practitioners experienced in these procedures. Challenge can be performed by oral, nasal, conjunctival or bronchial routes.

Radiology

The quality of information available from conventional x-rays of paranasal sinuses does not justify its use and CT scanning is the preferred procedure.

Chest x-ray should always be performed in acute asthma to exclude a number of conditions such as pneumothorax (which can be easily missed because of reduced breath sounds), infection, collapse or inhalation of a foreign body in a child.

Endoscopy

Rhinoscopy has added a new dimension to clinical practice. Experienced operators can perform the technique with a minimum of discomfort and an excellent picture can be obtained in a very short space of time. It is best considered a specialist procedure since interpretation requires frequent performance. Initially it was indicated in complicated cases and for excluding granulomatous conditions and malignancies, but it is now considered to be useful in all but the most straightforward and mildest cases of nasal disease.

Indications for bronchoscopy are to exclude a foreign body or tumour, or to obtain a lung biopsy.

Laboratory investigation

Laboratory tests are most useful when applied as indicated by clinical enquiry. In isolation they can be extremely misleading. They have three broad applications:

1. To confirm the presence of atopy

Total IgE measurement

In contrast to other immunoglobulin isotypes which are present in serum in amounts of g/L, IgE is present only in nanogram amounts and hence requires sensitive radioactive or enzyme linked systems for quantitation. Furthermore, there are a number of problems with interpretation:

(a) IgE is distributed in normal populations in a non-parametric manner, with a long 'tail' of high values. This makes it inappropriate to define a normal range based on mean ± 2 standard deviations or 95% confidence limits which are the usual practice for most analytes.

(b) Race, gender and age influence normal levels and these factors are often not taken into account. Serum IgE levels tend to be lower in Europe, North America and Australia, and higher in populations from underdeveloped countries.

(c) Genetic factors contribute to serum levels. To a degree this reflects inheritance of the atopic diathesis, but the presence of high levels does not necessarily equate with the presence of allergic disease.

Serum IgE levels are elevated to the greatest extent in atopic eczema, less so in asthma, and many patients with allergic rhinitis have normal levels, making it of limited diagnostic value in this condition.

Indications for total IgE are to determine whether an acute allergic reaction has occurred; distinguish allergic from infective bronchiolitis in children; assist in diagnosis of allergic bronchopulmonary aspergillosis; identify the allergic diathesis; assist in diagnosis of some rare immunodeficiency diseases; and indicate the presence of parasitic infestation.

It has been suggested that cord blood IgE levels are valuable in predicting the development of atopic disease in neonates, especially when performed in high risk situations such as when both parents are atopic. Elevated levels provide further incentives for preventative measures to be undertaken. Serum IgE levels maintain the same rank order as cord blood in infants up to nine months of age and are not affected by maternal smoking or other prenatal influences on IgE levels. Cord blood and infant levels are very low and the laboratory procedures require special modifications for measurement in this age group.

Multi-allergen diagnosis of atopy (Phadiatop[R] or Omnidisc[R])

This commercial technology was introduced to apply a large number of individual allergens to a single solid phase and to perform a RAST-type study. It is claimed to indicate atopy with more precision than total serum IgE, since the aggregate of multiple IgE specificities is measured instead of total IgE. These tests will answer the question whether patients are atopic, but not to which allergens they are allergic.

2. To demonstrate specific IgE antibodies (RAST)

There are now a number of laboratory procedures for the identification of allergen specific IgE antibody in serum. The term 'RAST' is used colloquially as the abbreviation for RadioAllergoSorbent Test. This was the original commercially developed methodology, although other technologies are now used to detect these antibodies, and other acronyms apply as well, such as EASTs (EnzymeAllergoSorbent Test).

RASTs provide similar information to skin prick tests. The agreement between RAST and SPT should theoretically be 100%. It approaches this if the same antigen is used and the patient shows a high degree of sensitivity. However, in the real world it is less than this. In most instances different allergens are used for skin prick testing and for RAST. The discrepancy between SPT and RAST is particularly marked with complex allergens such as mould extracts, where the concordance rate is in the order of 50%. Skin prick tests are more sensitive than RAST, although with modern technology, using the CAP® system, in vitro tests reach a similar degree of sensitivity.

RASTs have certain advantages in relation to convenience, cost and usage, in that they are easily standardised, there is little operator variability, they are not influenced by medication or skin disease, they are completely safe, and serum can be stored.

Their disadvantages are that technical factors can lead to false negatives when very high levels of specific IgG antibody are present which occupy allergen sites on the solid phase, and can lead to false positives from high levels of total IgE trapped on the solid phase non-specifically. These problems have largely been overcome with newer technology. They are more expensive than SPT and the number of allergens that can be tested for on each occasion of service is limited by the Medicare rebate.

Advantages of SPT include greater sensitivity than RASTs, lower cost if many patients are to be tested and immediate availability of results at the time of consultation. This is not only a convenience for patient and doctor but, more importantly, a reaction has a positive impact on management. Disadvantages are that the doctor has to maintain a range of solutions which may prove to be expensive if only a limited number of patients are to be tested.

RASTs are indicated in preference to skin tests when the patient is receiving antihistamines and especially astemizole (Hismanal); if there is widespread skin disease such as eczema which makes it difficult to find an area of normal skin; in the presence of dermatographism when there is non-specific reactivity to the trauma of the needle prick; in young children who may be frightened by the multiple punctures of skin tests; if the allergens are not available; and where skin testing may be dangerous, for example testing with insect venom or latex.

For the diagnosis of penicillin allergy the reagents for skin testing are not readily available and RASTs are more convenient but less sensitive. Skin testing for bee venom allergy should only be done in a hospital setting by experienced practitioners.

In a bid to reduce the number of allergens examined, manufacturers have batched several allergens on a single disc or solid phase. Performance appears to be equivalent to use of single allergens. There are several new technologies for detection of RAST, including the CAP® system. Some of these have advantages such as increased sensitivity.

3. *To determine the presence of an allergic reaction*

Measurement of mediators

Mediators can be measured in the serum or body fluids, or their releasability from cells can be determined when they are challenged with allergen in vitro. At present these investigations are still in the realms of clinical research, or are available only in special allergy units.

Histamine is a relatively unstable analyte and difficult to measure in the small amounts found in blood. Serum histamine levels rise in cold-induced urticaria and play a role in the hypotension and collapse which may accompany this condition. Levels are not usually elevated in other allergic conditions. Histamine may be measured in tissue culture following the incubation of cells from allergic subjects with the relevant allergen.

Tryptase is released from secretory granules of mast cells and can be measured in the serum in anaphylactic reactions with peak levels in 1 to 2 hours after an initial delay of 15 to 30 minutes. Levels remain elevated for up to 6 hours. Histamine levels in contrast, peak in 5 to 10 minutes and are back to baseline in 15 to 60 minutes. Furthermore, tryptase is relatively stable in serum and is unaffected by freezing and thawing. This makes it much more practical to measure than histamine. Elevated levels provide a valuable indication that an anaphylactic reaction has occurred. Situations where this might apply are in identifying the nature of reactions to bee sting or bee venom immunotherapy or during anaesthesia. Elevated levels can be found in post-mortem blood, which makes the test of considerable forensic importance in excluding anaphylaxis as a cause of sudden or unexpected death. There is some evidence that it is less reliable when the anaphylactic reaction has been induced by an ingestant.

Leukotrienes. A new technique (CAST-Elisa®) is now available in laboratory kit form for measuring release of leukotrienes from peripheral blood leucocytes incubated with the allergen. This procedure holds promise of providing more meaningful information about clinically important allergic reactions. RAST and SPT measure levels of specific IgE antibody and hence sensitisation, rather than indicating whether the allergens induce an allergic reaction. Its drawback is that it requires special laboratory facilities, and its place is likely to be in the investigation of particularly involved problems.

Cytology of secretions

Cytology of nasal secretions can be helpful in determining the nature of rhinitis. Typically allergic rhinitis is associated with clumps of eosinophils, while in infective rhinitis, large numbers of neutrophils are present. In NARES (non-allergic rhinitis with eosinophils), eosinophils are numerous, yet there is no obvious allergic basis for the symptoms. Counting of the cells can be misleading because of clumping of eosinophils and a descriptive interpretation of the findings is required.

Eosinophils and eosinophil products

It has long been appreciated that peripheral blood eosinophilia is an indicator of severity of asthma rather than that allergic factors are operative. More recently measurements have been made of eosinophil products such as ECP and EXP. ECP levels correlate with severity of asthma but their exact role in management remains to be determined.

Unproven diagnostic procedures

There are a number of procedures which are still used in diagnosis of allergy but which have no scientific validity. These include the demonstration of Candida-precipitating antibodies and circulating Candida organisms in the so-called Candida hypersensitivity syndrome, Bryan's cytotoxicity testing, the Alcat test and the Vega machine.

Further reading

Walls RS. Common Sense Pathology Unit 13: Allergy Testing. Pathology Education Committee, Royal Australasian Colleges of General Practitioners and of Pathologists, Sydney, November 1990.

Walls RS. Diagnosing allergies—the hows and whys. *Australian Family Physician* 1993; 22: 1937–43.

Chapter 3

Approach to management of allergic diseases

Aims

The aim of management in allergic diseases is to prevent progression of disease and the development of complications, and to improve quality of life. Quality of life (QOL) issues are assuming much greater importance in care of these patients. Formal QOL measures are being included more extensively in trials of new drugs, but it is becoming clear that they should also be used in management of individual patients. Good doctors consider these issues intuitively. However, in future years it will become increasingly important to consider these issues more formally. A greater array of effective treatments is becoming available, the long-term effects of which cannot be known. Nevertheless, they carry important implications for future health, especially in the younger age group who are mainly affected by allergic diseases which are chronic and whose manifestations are often intermittent. QOL assessment requires the use of tools to measure the effects of illness and of its treatment on the capacity of patients to function effectively, as perceived by themselves. Effects on physical and occupational activities, and on psychological, social and somatic factors are taken into account. These parameters may not correlate well with physiological measures and other traditional indications of disease severity. They need to be taken into account in designing the most appropriate overall management for the patient.

A graded approach to the management of allergic diseases is required because they vary widely in their severity, and in the mildest forms it may not be appropriate to progress to the more aggressive forms of treatment. The steps are outlined below but how they pertain to individual diseases is discussed more fully in the relevant chapters.

Allergen avoidance

Identification of the allergens responsible for provoking the allergic reaction and the initiation of measures to reduce exposure to them, forms the basis of all successful management programs. Patients need to be persuaded that these are an essential part of their management, and that drugs and desensitisation are not substitutes which allow them to escape from their responsibility to institute effective allergen avoidance measures.

TABLE 3.1 **A step-wise approach to management**

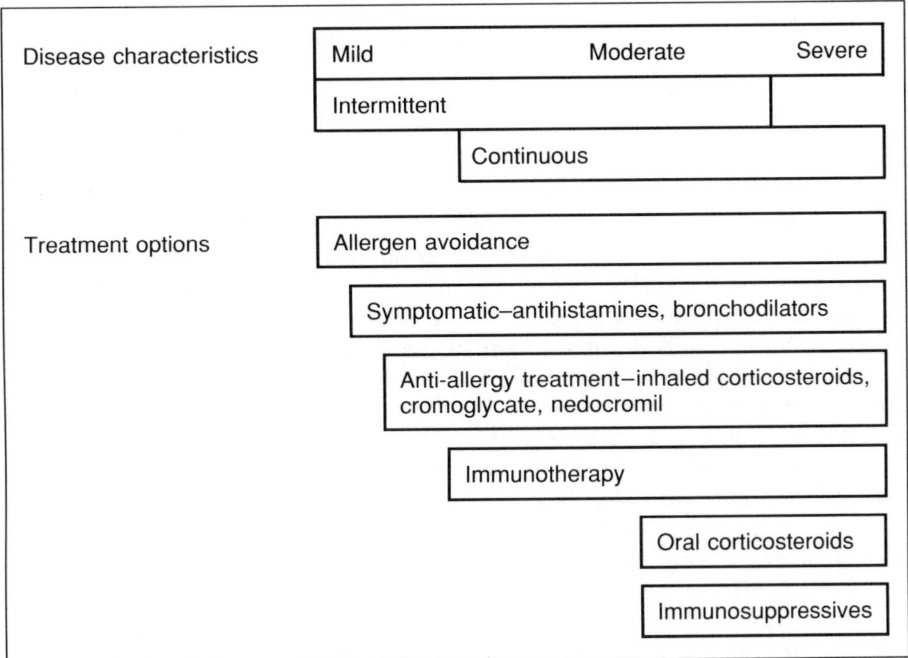

In the case of *house dust mite* allergy there is good evidence that strict measures to reduce exposure are effective in reducing symptoms and reversing bronchial hyperresponsiveness. Dust mite avoidance requires physical cleaning of the home environment (also the work or school environment if possible), and removal of dust traps such as fluffy toys. A good quality vacuum cleaner is important with adequate filtration of the exhaust air to ensure that allergen is not disseminated in the atmosphere. Bedding should be washed frequently in water hotter than 65°C and aired in the sun or dried at high temperatures in clothes driers. Carpets and soft furnishings can be treated with miticides which are based on benzyl-benzoate or tannate. Insecticides are not effective against dust mites.

It may be necessary to deny the *cat or other pet* access to the house or to find another home for it. Even though the pet has been removed from the environment, the allergens remain in furnishings for long periods afterwards and can cause symptoms.

Avoidance of pollens is more difficult to achieve. Patients are affected only during the pollen season, providing natural proof that lack of exposure leads to improvement in symptoms. Certain simple measures can assist in reducing pollen exposure. These include avoiding high pollen areas such as farms, staying indoors with windows closed and using an air-conditioner during the pollen season. Subjects should drive with car windows closed and the air-conditioner on. It is helpful to wear glasses outdoors to assist in protecting the eyes. Lawns should be mowed frequently to avoid flowering, and it is helpful to wear a mask if the patient has to perform this function. Garden plants which are low pollen producers should be selected. These are usually the native species.

Fungi and moulds are ubiquitous and less is known about their behaviour. There are indoor and outdoor species, both of which can precipitate allergies. Open compost heaps should be avoided and fallen leaves and garden debris removed. Indoor mould can be reduced by good ventilation, ensuring the house is in good repair and treatment of damp.

Good building design and construction is also important in reducing house dust mite growth. There was a great increase in house dust mite allergy in Europe following the energy crisis in 1974 due to a change in construction methods designed to ensure a tight seal with a minimum of air exchange to conserve warmth. Indoor humidity rose and the house dust mite population increased dramatically, leading to an increase in asthma. Modern designs are starting to take cognisance of the problem. Houses need to be built to ensure adequate ventilation and to minimise humidity and dampness. Low humidity is difficult to achieve in tropical and subtropical climates, even with air-conditioning. There should be no dust traps such as pelmets and thick drapes, and smooth floors without carpeting are preferred.

Identification of *offending foods* is a difficult exercise which relies heavily on elimination and provocation procedures. Once identified, a suitable diet must be designed which excludes the component responsible for symptoms. This requires professional dietary management since the treatment is longstanding, and great harm can be done from inadequate nutrition, especially in children.

General health measures

General health measures and physical fitness are important in chronic diseases such as allergy. Asthma camps fulfil a valuable role and exercise improves physiological function. The psychological effects of a sense of well-being are beneficial for these diseases, and biological mechanisms are being explored in the laboratory to explain this phenomenon.

Symptomatic treatment

Where symptoms are mild and intermittent it may be sufficient for the patient to take symptomatic treatment, including antihistamines, topical or oral adrenergic decongestants and β-2 agonists such as salbutamol.

Anti-inflammatory and preventive therapy

With more persistent and severe disease it is usually necessary to prescribe preventive therapy which is anti-inflammatory and anti-allergic. The newer second generation antihistamines have demonstrable anti-allergic properties in experimental situations but their importance in the clinical context is not yet clear. Inhaled corticosteroids are our most effective anti-inflammatory agents at present and they should be prescribed early in the natural history of the disease to control inflammation, reduce hyperresponsiveness of target organs and prevent disease progression. Sodium cromoglycate is an efficient and safe anti-inflammatory agent especially in children. Nedocromil sodium fulfils a similar function in moderate asthma.

Immunosuppressive agents have been used in severe disease. At one time gold was prescribed for severe asthma, but more recently success has been claimed for methotrexate and cyclosporin A in refractory asthmatics, and methotrexate and azathioprine have been used in severe atopic eczema.

Immunological treatment

Despite its many imperfections and drawbacks, immunotherapy is the only treatment available at present which is capable of modifying the disease process in a permanent or prolonged fashion. Because it requires a significant investment in time and carries some risks it should be considered after other measures have been instituted, where there is the likelihood of success (before secondary pathological changes have occurred) and where an allergen can be clearly identified as contributing significantly to the pathological process.

Further reading

Breslin ABX. New developments in anti-asthma drugs. *Med J Aust* 1993; 158: 779–82.

Juniper EF, Guyatt GH, Dolovich J. Assessment of quality of life in adolescents with allergic conjunctivitis: development and testing of a questionnaire for clinical trials. *J Allergy Clin Immunol* 1994; 93: 413–23.

Tovey E (ed). Mites, asthma and domestic design II. The University Printing Service, University of Sydney, 1995.

Chapter 4

Inhalational therapy

Delivery of drugs by inhalation has largely replaced systemic administration for respiratory allergies in all but a few indications such as anaphylaxis, respiratory obstruction from angioedema and severe bronchospasm. The advantages are that the drug is delivered directly to the affected target tissue so that a smaller dose is required with more efficient utilisation and less opportunity for systemic side effects. Effective doses of oral salbutamol produce plasma levels in the order of 5 to 15 ng/ml in contrast to levels of far less than 1 ng/ml with inhaled drug.

Methods of administration

An ideal inhalational device has not yet been developed. The particle size generated by the device is the most important variable determining the site of deposition of aerosol in the respiratory tract. Other important variables are the rate of inhalation, whether administered through nose or mouth, and factors which influence evaporation and condensation of aerosols such as solubility of drug, and whether the vehicle is water, solvent or dry powder. Deposition in alveoli is optimal with particle sizes around 2 to 3 microns at slow rates of inhalation (20 to 30 L/min). Breath-holding after inhalation also tends to increase deposition of particles in distal airways. Distribution in asthmatics tends to be more central than in normal subjects because of bronchoconstriction which affects the terminal bronchioles and prevents access of aerosols to the the more distal, poorly ventilated alveoli. Delivery systems in current usage are:

1. *Metered dose inhalers* (MDI). A propellant discharges a metered volume when the device is actuated, and the patient is required to co-ordinate his respiratory effort to inhale the discharged suspension. Particle sizes are larger than ideal and a significant proportion of the drug impacts on the oropharynx. Shaking the canister before use is important to disperse the drug in the solvents which are formulated to reduce surface tension and stabilise the suspension. Although only minute amounts of chlorofluorocarbon (CFC) propellant are discharged, the ecological concerns are ensuring that ultimately alternative delivery systems will be used.

   The degree of co-ordination required is not always sufficient, especially in the young and the old. To overcome this problem spacers and reservoirs have been designed which provide extra time between discharge and inhalation to allow for droplet evaporation reducing aerosol particle size, retaining some of the larger particles, reducing velocity, and therefore reducing the likelihood of impaction in the upper airways. With spacers, inhalation coincides with activation. Reservoirs are larger and actuation takes place before inhalation. There is far less requirement for co-ordination with these devices and they are therefore especially useful for the very young and the old.

2. *Dry powder generators.* These devices aerosolise a set dose of drug in micronised powder form. Delivery depends on the patient's own respiratory effort and does not require the same degree of co-ordination as MDI's. The first of these were single-dose inhalers represented by the Spinhaler® for sodium cromoglycate. More recently multidose devices, the Turbuhaler® for delivery of budesonide and terbutaline and the Diskhaler® have become available, using the same principle. Patients need to inhale rapidly, in excess of 60 L/min, to activate these devices.

3. *Nebulizers (Air-blast nebulizers).* Air or oxygen is passed through the therapeutic solution causing a mist which is then inhaled through a mask. This is the most reliable form of administration and is used in children and for acute exacerbations of asthma in hospital. It is generally agreed that a higher dose is achieved than with MDI, particle sizes are less than 5 microns, and there is good lung penetration. A 3 ml volume of 0.83 mg/ml solution of salbutamol results in more than ten times the amount reaching the lungs than from two puffs from an MDI.

Drugs administered by inhalation

β-2 agonists

These are effective bronchodilators, valuable for relief of symptoms and for treatment of exacerbations where at times they are life-saving. Modern drugs are highly selective, although in some patients larger doses can lead to palpitations, tremor and agitation. Earlier recommendations were for these drugs to be used on a regular basis. However, there has been a re-examination of their role following reports which suggested that some preparations were associated with increased asthma mortality. There are suggestions that their regular use results in worse asthma control, that tolerance may develop to bronchodilator and bronchoprotective effects, especially with the long-acting preparations, and that there may be an increase in bronchial hyper-responsiveness and increased allergen-induced airway inflammation with their use. Practice with these agents has changed. It is now advised that these drugs be used on an 'as required' basis for symptomatic relief. Increasing requirements are an indication that asthma is getting out of control and an indication for more intensive anti-inflammatory therapy such as increased inhaled corticosteroids. Beta-2 agonists have no anti-inflammatory properties. Long-acting preparations such as salmeterol and formoterol should not be used for relief of acute asthma. Their main current indication is for frequent nocturnal asthma despite maximum doses of inhaled corticosteroids.

Corticosteroids

These drugs now form the mainstay of treatment of asthma in all but the mildest cases. They are anti-inflammatory and can be shown to reduce bronchial inflammation on serial biopsy. They therefore modify the disease process. The same principles apply to their use as to that of corticosteroids in other situations. Initially a high dose should be used to obtain control, and after 4 to 8 weeks it is reduced to a maintenance which will keep the patient symptom-free. Doses of beclomethasone under 1,600 mcg per day in adults, under 600 mcg per day in children under 5, and under 1,000 mcg per day in older children are considered safe. If nasal steroids are used at the same time the dosage must be taken into account in calculating the total daily dosage. In children, and with the use of large doses in adults, a spacer device should be used to minimise the risk of local toxicity.

Administration. Careful explanation and demonstration of how to use the various devices should always be given, and technique should be checked on return visits until the doctor is satisfied that it is satisfactory. After each dosage patients should gargle and rinse their mouths to reduce the likelihood of oropharyngeal candidiasis. The liquid should be spat out rather than swallowed to reduce gastro-intestinal absorption.

Side effects of inhaled corticosteroids are oropharyngeal candidiasis, hoarse voice, and evidence of systemic absorption with easy bruising which occurs with large doses. Inhaled corticosteroids should not be relied on for control of acute asthma. Under these circumstances systemic corticosteroids are indicated.

Sodium cromoglycate

This drug is free of side effects and is an effective anti-inflammatory agent and preventative in asthma. It is the drug of first choice in children with mild to moderate asthma, and is useful in some adults as a substitute for inhaled corticosteroids or as a steroid-sparing agent. It is effective in preventing exercise-induced asthma in both adults and children when used about 15 minutes before starting to exercise. Its onset of action is slow and 4 weeks of therapy should be undertaken before deciding on its efficacy. It should be administered three to four times daily initially, a disadvantage when compared with inhaled corticosteroids, although twice a day may be sufficient for maintenance therapy. It can be delivered by MDI, Spinhaler® dry powder generator or by nebuliser. Although in use for over 25 years its mode of action is still not clear. It was originally introduced as a mast cell stabilising agent but more effective agents have been introduced subsequently and found not to be as effective in management of asthma. One recent suggestion is that it may function as a tachykinin antagonist.

Nedocromil sodium

This drug belongs to a new class of compound, the pyranoquinolines. In vitro it suppresses the activity of inflammatory cells and inhibits tachykinin pathways. It is effective in mild to moderate asthma and is useful as an inhaled steroid sparing agent. It also appears to be effective in suppressing the cough in patients with asthma, following viral infections and possibly due to ACE inhibitors, although it is not approved for use in the latter two conditions. Side effects are infrequent and not severe, the most troublesome being an unpleasant bitter taste in 12% of patients. From 5–7% of patients describe nausea or vomiting, sore throat, cough or headache.

Ipratropium bromide

This is an anticholinergic agent which has a complementary role to inhaled β-2 agonists in some patients, especially those with an element of chronic bronchitis and excessive mucoid secretions. It may be helpful in postviral cough and cough variant asthma.

Further reading

Barnes PJ, Pedersen S. Efficacy and safety of inhaled corticosteroids in asthma. *Am Rev Respir Dis* 1993; 148: S1–26.

Byron PR. Inhalation devices. *In:* D'Arcy PF, McElnay JC (eds). The Pharmacology and Pharmacotherapy of Asthma. Chichester, UK: Ellis Horwood, 1968; 137–59.

Cockcroft DW, McParland CP, Britto SA, Swystun VA, Rutherford BC. Regular inhaled salbutamol and airway responsiveness to allergen. *Lancet* 1993; 342: 833–7. (See also Britton J. Editorial. *Lancet* 1993; 342: 818–9).

Edwards AM, Stevens MT. The clinical efficacy of nedocromil sodium (Tilade) in the treatment of asthma. *Eur Respir J* 1993; 6: 35–41.

Chapter 5

Antihistamines

Antihistamines have been available to medical practice for around 50 years. They are widely used and most are now available as non-prescription, over the counter (OTC) preparations. As a group they have a good safety record.

In 1910 Dale was the first to show that histamine was able to induce a shock-like syndrome when injected into animals. Further work established its importance as a mediator of allergic reactions in man. Histamine has proved to be but one of many mediators, a major player in allergic events in the nose and skin, but of less importance in the bronchi. As expected, antihistamines are less effective in asthma. In 1966 Ash and Schild suggested that there was a second type of histamine receptor, and in 1972 Black confirmed that stimulation of these H2 receptors was responsible for acid secretion in the stomach. The classical antihistamines have no effect on H2 receptors and a different group of drugs were developed which include cimetidine, ranitidine and famotidine, devoid of anti-allergy properties (except in chronic urticaria where concomitant blockade of H1 and H2 receptors can be more effective in some patients than blockade of H1 receptors alone). A third class of histamine receptor, the H3 receptor, occurs in the brain and has a negative modulating function.

The first clinically useful antihistamines became available by the mid-1940s. Many of the early drugs were relatively weak and large doses were required for their antihistamine effects, so that their other pharmacological activities became obtrusive. Diphenhydramine was introduced in 1946 and remains in clinical use to this day, being one of the few preparations available in this country for intravenous use.

A large number of drugs came on to the market over the succeeding years, belonging to different chemical classes. To a greater or lesser extent they were all sedating. The big breakthrough came in the early 1980s with the development of highly specific H1 blocking agents which were devoid of sedative properties.

Pharmacology

Histamine is a simple amine with a ring nucleus and a side chain (Fig 5.1). The H1 blocking agents resemble the side chain in chemical structure while H2 blocking agents mimic the ring nucleus. The distribution of these receptors determines their function.

FIGURE 5.1 Chemical structure of histamine and some antihistamines.

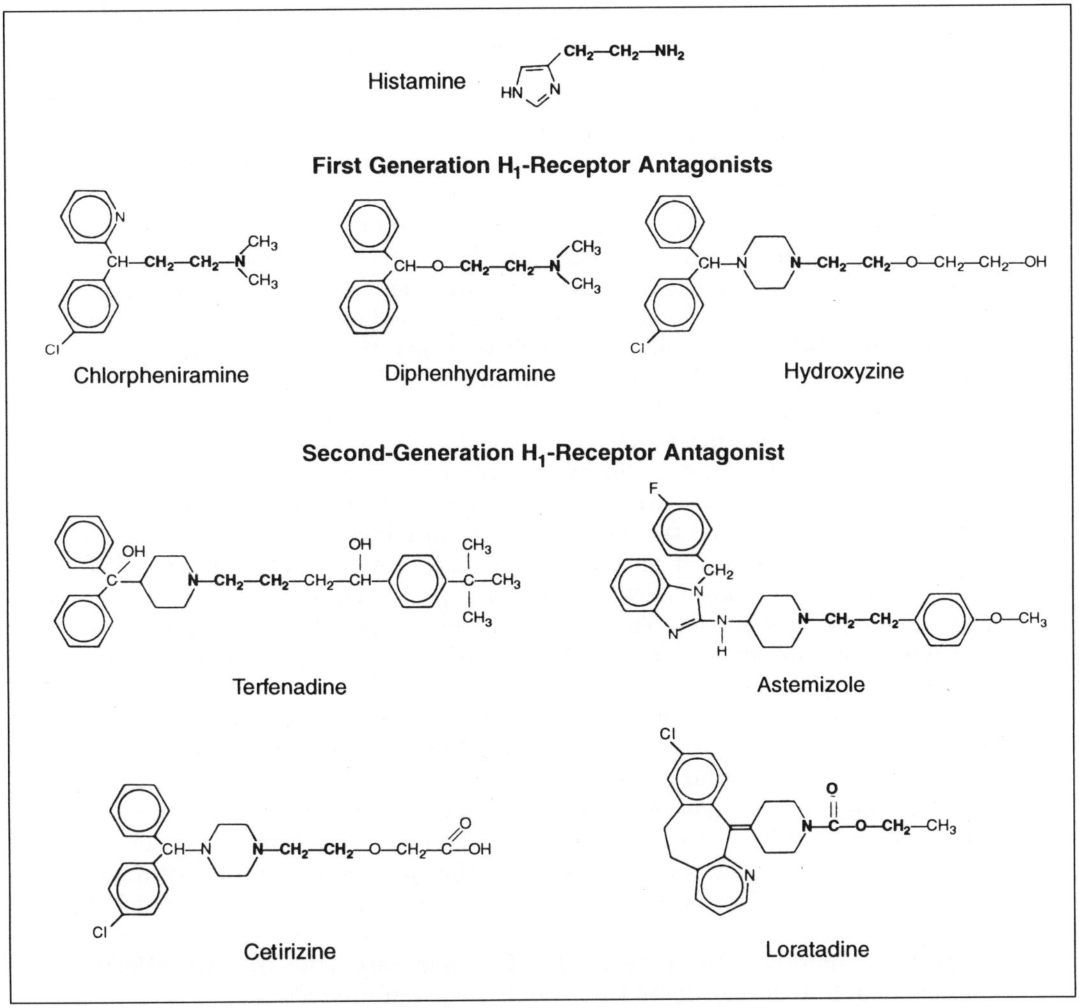

Histamine

First Generation H₁-Receptor Antagonists

Chlorpheniramine

Diphenhydramine

Hydroxyzine

Second-Generation H₁-Receptor Antagonist

Terfenadine

Astemizole

Cetirizine

Loratadine

TABLE 5.1 Effects of histamine H1 and H2 stimulation

H1 receptor	Vascular permeability
	Smooth muscle contraction
	Sensory nerve stimulation with pruritus
	Vagal stimulation in airways
	Prostaglandin and neuropeptide generation
H2 receptor	Gastric acid secretion
	Increased mucus secretion in airways
	Negative feedback on basophil histamine release
	Suppresses lymphocyte function
	Inhibits neutrophil and monocyte function

Antihistamines are competitive inhibitors of H1 receptors. They are readily displaced and so tend to have a short duration of action. Newer H1 blocking agents are both competitive and non-competitive antagonists of H1 receptors, therefore dissociating more slowly and having a longer duration of action. Since antihistamines compete with histamine for its receptor, they are most effective when given before allergen exposure. Larger doses are required to displace histamine from its receptor.

Antihistamines belong to several different families of chemical substances, and in the case of the first generation drugs, their antihistaminic properties are but one of several pharmacological properties which include muscarinic, anticholinergic, adrenergic and local anaesthetic effects. Drugs in one chemical family tend to have similar properties. It used to be important to be familiar with drugs from several classes to enable one to avoid, or make use of, some of their other pharmacological actions. However, second generation agents are highly selective H1 antagonists and are largely free of other pharmacological properties.

Responses to individual drugs vary widely between subjects in a way which is difficult to predict, so the availability of a number of different agents is important. Some have particular properties which favour their use in specific situations, but on the whole they are interchangeable.

The clinical efficacy of antihistamines does not correlate directly with their histamine receptor blockade in vitro, partly because of their other pharmacological properties. The anticholinergic properties of a drug such as chlorpheniramine can be a very useful adjunct for drying nasal secretions. Several of the newer drugs have been shown to have other anti-allergic properties. Some can be shown to decrease the release of mediators from cells during antigen challenge, including the lipid-derived mediators such as the leukotrienes. Some inhibit cell adhesion molecule function, important in cell mobility and the inflammatory response, and cetirizine reduces the accumulation of eosinophils in inflammatory foci. To the extent that H1 receptor blockade does not offer the whole explanation for the action of antihistamines, they are perhaps best considered as anti-allergy drugs with major H1 receptor blockade effects. The clinical significance of these other anti-allergy properties remains to be determined. In some cases the in vitro effects require relatively larger doses than would be given in vivo.

The advent of the newer antihistamines has been a significant therapeutic advance. They cause little or no sedation, they have a higher specificity for peripheral histamine receptors than those in the central nervous system and lack other pharmacological effects such as anticholinergic and muscarinic properties. Several are derivatives of classical drugs, for example loratadine from azatadine, and cetirizine from hydroxyzine. Others such as astemizole do not belong to any of the previous chemical families. Tachyphylaxis or tolerance to antihistaminic effects does not occur with long-term administration of these agents.

Suppression of the wheal induced by intradermal injection of histamine gives a reliable indication of the biological effects of the antihistamines. It is necessary to bear this in mind when performing diagnostic skin prick testing with allergens. It is sufficient to stop most drugs 48 hours before testing, but

TABLE 5.2 **Some H1 receptor blocking agents**

Class	Generic Name	Comments
Ethanolamine		Sedation, anticholinergic effects common. Low incidence of gastro-intestinal side effects
	Clemastine	
	Diphenhydramine	Available for IV injection
	Dimenhydrinate	Used for motion sickness, nausea
	Diphenylpyraline	
Alkylamines	Phenyramine	Sedation less common, except at high dosage. CNS stimulation may occur
	Bromphenyramine	
	Chlorpheniramine	
	Dexchlorpheniramine	
	Triprolidine	
Ethylenediamines	Clemizole	Topical use liable to produce sensitisation, especially on abnormal skin
	Mepyramine	
Phenothiazines		Sedating and anticholinergic; some used as anti-emetics and for sedation
	Promethazine HCl	Available for injection
	Trimeprazine	
	Methdilazine	
	Promethazine theoclate	Used for motion sickness
Piperazines	Hydroxyzine	Useful in urticaria
	Mebhydrolin	Reversible agranulocytosis and neutropenia reported rarely
	Cetirizine	Low-sedating, potent
Piperidines	Terfenadine	Non-sedating
	Azatadine	Unlikely to sedate
	Cyproheptadine	Useful in cold urticaria
	Loratadine	Non-sedating
Other	Astemizole	Non-sedating; long half-life
	Levocabastine	Topically active

in the case of astemizole the wheal is inhibited for 4 to 6 weeks, and some suppression of wheal and flare responses may still be observed even 14 weeks after stopping the drug in some patients. This characteristic effectively precludes skin testing in patients receiving this drug. The duration of wheal suppression is dose-dependent. For example, 60 mg of terfenadine suppresses the wheal response for 12 hours, but two tablets (120 mg) suppresses the response for 24 hours.

As with all drugs, use of antihistamines should be avoided wherever possible in pregnancy, although none have been linked with an increased incidence of human fetal malformations or irreversible damage.

Absorption and metabolism

Antihistamines are well absorbed by mouth, although it has been claimed that absorption of astemizole is reduced in the presence of food.

Terfenadine, astemizole and loratadine undergo extensive first-pass metabolism in the liver and are rapidly changed to active compounds so that peak serum concentrations of the native drugs are extremely low. The first two drugs use the P450 cytochrome oxidase enzyme system, so that co-administration of other drugs which also are metabolised by that pathway result in their accumulation. The situation with terfenadine has been particularly well studied. It has been shown that the parent compound has quinidine-like properties, leading to conduction disturbances. Loratidine is also extensively metabolised in the liver, although not through the P450 cytochrome pathway. Nonetheless, it accumulates in the presence of impaired liver function, and the result of this extensive hepatic metabolism on vulnerability to co-administration of drugs metabolised by P450 is not yet entirely clear. Ketoconazole, which is one such drug, decreases loratadine elimination. Cetirizine is the active metabolite of hydroxyzine and is not metabolised further to a significant degree in humans. It is excreted largely unchanged in the urine so that its half-life is increased to about 18 hours in patients with renal failure. One interaction study so far of cetirizine with cimetidine has shown no decrease in elimination.

The active metabolite of terfenadine, terfenadine acid metabolite (TAM) or fexofenadine, has been submitted for marketing approval in several countries. Like cetirizine it does not undergo any significant metabolism and is excreted largely in the faeces. This agent is free of the quinidine-like effects of the parent compound.

The serum half-life of several drugs is age-dependent. Terfenadine, for example, is cleared more rapidly in children and more slowly in the elderly.

Of the newer agents not yet marketed, ebastine is metabolised by the cytochrome P450 pathway, while acrivastine, which is a topically active antihistamine, is excreted largely unchanged. Levocabastine and acrivastine are new topically active antihistamines. Both are sedating when used systemically.

Which antihistamine?

First or second generation drug?

The first decision is whether there is any longer a role for first generation drugs. Sales figures for antihistamines in Australia show that first generation agents still account for a significant proportion of sales, although second generation antihistamines are becoming the first choice to an increasing degree because they lack CNS-depressant properties. The second generation agents are highly selective H1 blocking agents and lack many other pharmacological properties. This may be a disadvantage in some circumstances where the 'unwanted' effects of older drugs may be useful. For example, anticholinergic properties of drugs such as chlorpheniramine may assist in control of symptoms such as nasal secretion in some patients. The anxiolytic properties of hydroxyzine are particularly useful in chronic urticaria.

Sedative effects of first generation drugs are highly individual and there is no way of predicting with certainty how a particular patient will react. It may be possible to dissociate the sedative from the antihistamine properties by:

(a) reducing the dose. Some patients derive sufficient antihistaminic benefit from paediatric dosages without the sedation usually associated with the full adult dose;

(b) giving the drug at night so that the resulting somnolence occurs during the sleeping hours, while the H1 receptor blockade persists through the next day. There is evidence, however, that impaired CNS function may exist in the absence of symptoms. With dust mite allergy, the night hours are often the times of maximal exposure to allergen in the domestic environment;

(c) trying another drug, especially from a different chemical class;

(d) continuing the drug so that tolerance to the side effects occurs. This is not always successful.

Use of agents which are potentially sedating when alternatives are available without this problem has possible medico-legal implications. Such situations are likely to arise in driving a motor vehicle, operating machinery, or even when a clear mind is required. There is epidemiological evidence that first generation H1 antagonists are implicated in fatal traffic accidents.

One disadvantage of the newer agents is that they are more expensive, and when this is a consideration it is nearly always possible to use one of the older drugs in a way which reduces these problems significantly. Another approach is to use a first generation drug at night and a second generation agent such as terfenadine, which has a 12 hour duration of action, in the mornings.

Which second generation antihistamine?

Four are currently available in Australia, namely terfenadine, astemizole, loratidine and cetirizine. There is little difference in efficacy between these drugs, although there is considerable individual variability in responses, and some patients may respond better to one than to another.

New work is starting to define histamine receptors structurally as well as pharmacologically, and it is likely that there will be phenotypic variation in these receptors which will help to explain why certain chemical structures are more effective in some patients than others. Certainly minor structural changes in antagonist molecules can have profound effects on specific activity and by inference, on efficacy and safety. One agent that stands out for a different profile in its speed of onset and duration of action is astemizole. It may have some perceived advantages in chronic disorders such as chronic urticaria, but its long half-life precludes investigation by skin prick testing. Terfenadine is a truly non-sedating antihistamine even at high dosages, whereas loratadine may become sedating at higher doses and cetirizine makes some patients tired.

TABLE 5.3 **A comparison of second generation non-sedating antihistamines**

	Astemizole	Cetirizine	Loratadine	Terfenadine
Speed of onset	Slow	Rapid	Rapid	Rapid
Duration of action (elimination half-life of active metabolite)	9.5 days	7.5 hours	17 hours	17 hours
Dosage	10 mg Once daily	10 mg Once daily	10 mg Once daily	60 mg Twice daily
Timing requirements	Not with food	Nil	Nil	Nil
Wash-out period for skin testing	6 weeks	48 hours	48 hours	48 hours
Impaired performance	No	Slightly more than placebo	Nil at usual dose	No
Interaction with alcohol and benzodiazepines	Nil	Nil	Nil	Nil
May increase dosage	No	Yes*	Yes*	No
Weight gain	Possible	No	No	No

*may be sedating.

Clinical indications

As 'anti-allergic' drugs

Many allergic diseases present with multisystem involvement, and antihistamines then have decided advantages over the use of topical therapy at multiple sites, for example when treating rhinitis accompanied by conjunctivitis.

Rhinitis. Antihistamines are first line drugs, often used before medical attention is sought. They may be sufficient therapy alone, particularly for short-term use, but they are also valuable as ancillary agents together with topical corticosteroids. They are more effective in controlling sneezing, itching and rhinorrhoea than nasal obstruction, and are more effective in allergic than vasomotor rhinitis. Several preparations combine antihistamines with oral decongestants such as phenylephrine or pseudoephedrine, which are helpful in drying secretions and relieving obstruction. Care needs to be exercised with the use of these agents (see 'Side Effects' below).

Urticaria. Antihistamines are effective agents, but the dose may need to be increased to obtain effective receptor blockade. Antihistamines are less useful in angioedema. Some symptoms may persist despite complete H1 receptor blockade, implying that other mediators may also play a role in urticaria or that histamine may act through other receptors. Combination of an H1 blocking agent with an H2 agent such as cimetidine is more effective in some patients. It is difficult to predict which drug is likely to give the best results in an individual patient, but several drugs have particular value in certain situations. Cyproheptadine is especially useful in cold urticaria, and hydroxyzine in cholinergic urticaria. Hydroxyzine has mild anxiolytic properties and is often more effective in chronic urticaria than other agents. Doxepin, widely used as an antidepressant, also has potent antihistamine properties and may be successful in chronic urticaria when other agents have failed.

Anaphylaxis. In acute severe allergic reactions antihistamines are not first line drugs but they can be useful in controlling the associated urticaria. They are also useful to have at hand for patients who are allergic to insect stings. Oral suspensions are more rapidly absorbed than tablets and so are preferred, although they are less convenient to store. The only injectable antihistamines available in Australia are promethazine 25 mg/ml and diphenhydramine.

Eczema. Antihistamines have mild antipruritic effects and help the patient to control scratching. The sedative properties of the first generation drugs are beneficial, and hydroxyzine is particularly useful in eczema.

Asthma. It used to be taught that antihistamines were contra-indicated because of their tendency to dry secretions. However, it is becoming clearer now that they may be helpful for several reasons. Allergic rhinitis often accompanies asthma and may herald the onset of attacks or coincide with them, and asthma can be improved by attention to nasal symptoms for a number of reasons. Environmental factors such as pollens affect nose and lungs together. A naso-bronchial reflex has been postulated to explain why bronchospasm follows an allergic reaction in the nose. Some of the second generation drugs have anti-allergy properties apart from competitive blockade of histamine receptors and have been shown to possess mild anti-asthma properties.

In cold remedies

Antihistamines form part of the formulation of some popular mixtures of OTC drugs sold as anti-cold preparations, usually in association with an adrenergic agent such as pseudoephedrine, ephedrine or phenylephrine and an antipyretic/analgesic like paracetamol or aspirin. These mixtures have the potential for harmful side effects such as somnolence, provoking urinary retention where there is prostatism, or aggravating glaucoma. In practice, very few adverse reactions seem to be reported, given their common usage, but they should be avoided in patients at particular risk of toxicity.

As anti-emetics and antinauseants

Dimenhydrinate, diphenhydramine, cyclizine and promethazine are all used widely, either alone or in combination with hyoscine, to prevent motion sickness, in Ménière's syndrome, and combined with ergotamine in antimigraine preparations. Many are OTC preparations and precautions about sedation apply to them as to other antihistamines.

Sedation and premedication

Some antihistamines are used for their sedating properties, especially in children. These include promethazine and trimeprazine.

Topical applications

Levocabastine is a potent topical antihistamine which has recently become available for allergic rhinitis and conjunctivitis. It has comparable efficacy to topical corticosteroids. Promethazine and mepyramine have been formulated in ointments for use in symptomatic relief of minor itching, insect bites and minor burns, but sensitisation has been reported and their use in this way is not advisable.

Side effects and adverse reactions

The most noticeable difference between first and second generation drugs is in their side-effect profile. There is no evidence of dependency developing with any of the drugs.

Central nervous system. The major adverse reactions of the classical antihistamines is through their effects on the central nervous system, producing somnolence, sedation and drowsiness. They potentiate the effects of other CNS depressants such as alcohol. Patients should always be warned of the hazards of driving vehicles or operating machinery while taking antihistamines. CNS stimulation may also occur with some first generation drugs, resulting in hallucinations or convulsions in extreme cases when given in large doses. Children are particularly susceptible to these effects.

Careful studies have failed to show any effect of the newer drugs on driving skills or on psychomotor performance. However, in some clinical trials with cetirizine, subjective tiredness has been reported. No interaction has been shown between these drugs and alcohol or diazepam.

Anticholinergic properties. These occur to a varying degree in many of the classical antihistamines and lead to dry mouth and blurring of vision, urinary retention in the presence of prostatic hypertrophy, pyloroduodenal obstruction (due to stenosing peptic ulcer) and glaucoma. Drugs with pronounced anticholinergic properties should be avoided in patients with prostatic enlargement and with glaucoma. Second generation agents are highly specific for the H1 receptors and lack these side effects.

Cardiovascular toxicity. There has been considerable recent media coverage of the potential cardiotoxicity of terfenadine and astemizole. *Torsade de pointes* (TDP), a malignant tachyarrhythmia, syncope and cardiac arrest, has been reported rarely with astemizole, usually in the face of huge overdosage in the order of 200 mg or 20 times the recommended dose. Recently however, the Food and Drug Administration (FDA) in the United States has drawn attention to the fact that severe cardiac arrhythmias can be associated with this drug in doses from as little as 20 to 30 mg per day, only two to three times the recommended dose. In view of this, it is advised that the recommended dose of 10 mg per day should not be exceeded.

The situation with terfenadine has been studied in great detail. The parent compound is associated with quinidine-like effects and can prolong the QT interval and cause ventricular arrhythmias under certain circumstances. After the recommended dose the parent compound is present in plasma concentrations in the order of <10 mcg/L. However, these levels increase in conditions of interactions with other drugs which share the cytochrome P450 pathway in the liver. These include the macrolide antibiotics (erythromycin and congenors) and ketoconazole. Levels also increase in liver impairment, and other risk factors are patients with medical conditions leading to a prolonged QT interval such as hypokalaemia and the congenital QT syndrome. The terfenadine metabolite (terfenadine acid metabolite or fexofenadine) has no effect on the QT interval and is free of cardiotoxicity.

These effects need to be seen in perspective. They are exceedingly rare when taking into account the number of prescriptions for these agents dispensed worldwide, and with terfenadine have invariably occurred in the settings described above. A prospective community study showed no increase in the relative risk of developing cardiac toxicity while on terfenadine. A surprising finding, however, was an increase in cardiac events in subjects taking over-the-counter first generation antihistamines among which diphenhydramine was over-represented (Pratt et al, *Amer J Cardiol* 1994; 73: 346–52). Indeed, the Adverse Drug Reactions Advisory Council (ADRAC) of the Therapeutic Goods Administration in Australia has received more reports of arrhythmias related to loratidine than to terfenadine.

TABLE 5.4 Categorisation of risk of drug use in pregnancy

Category	Antihistamines classified
A	Meclozine, cyclizine, chlorcyclizine, hydroxyzine, brompheniramine, chlorpheniramine, clemastine, cyproheptadine, dexchlorpheniramine, diphenhydramine, diphenylamine, doxylamine, mebhydrolin, pheniramine, triprolidine
B_1	Loratadine
B_2	Azatadine, diphenylpyraline, methdilazine, terfenadine
C	Phenothiazines—promethazine, trimeprazine, (when given in high doses late in pregnancy prolonged extra-pyramidal disturbances have occurred in the child)
D	Levocabastine

A Drugs which have been taken by a large number of pregnant women and women of child-bearing age without an increase in frequency of malformations or other direct or indirect harmful effects on the fetus having been observed.

B Drugs which have been taken by only a limited number of pregnant women and women of child-bearing age without an increase in the frequency of malformation or other direct or indirect harmful effects on the human fetus having been observed. This is subcategorised on the basis of experience in animal studies:

B_1 No evidence of an increased occurrence of fetal damage

B_2 Studies inadequate and may be lacking, but available data shows no evidence of an increased occurrence of fetal damage

B_3 Evidence of increased occurrence of fetal damage, the significance of which is considered uncertain in humans.

C Drugs which, owing to their pharmacological effects, have caused or may be suspected of causing harmful effects on the human fetus or neonate without causing malformations. These effects may be reversible.

D Drugs which have caused an increased incidence of human fetal malformations or irreversible damage. These drugs may also have adverse pharmacological effects.

Source: *Medicines in Pregnancy*. Australian Drug Evaluation Committee, 2nd ed., 1992.

It should be remembered that cardiac effects have been reported with first generation antihistamines as well as tricyclic antidepressants. Tachycardia is not uncommon, due to the anticholinergic properties of the drugs. Diphenhydramine and hydroxyzine have been reported to cause adverse cardiovascular effects after large doses. Prolonged QT intervals and TDP have been reported with doxepin, imipramine and other tricyclic antidepressants with structural similarity to some H1 antagonists. Doxepin is a useful antihistamine clinically.

Other effects. Fever, gastro-intestinal disturbances and drug rashes have been reported infrequently. Headache, dizziness and hypertension are more likely to occur in the elderly. Increased appetite and weight gain has been reported in some patients with astemizole and cyproheptadine.

Combination preparations which include adrenergic agents as decongestants have additional hazards such as palpitations and other sympathomimetic side effects including insomnia, mydriasis, weakness and tachycardia. These combinations should be used with caution in patients with a history of hypertension, narrow angle glaucoma, coronary artery disease, hyperthyroidism or prostatic hypertrophy.

Sensitisation can occur when these drugs are used topically.

Reactions to colouring agents and excipients. Not all adverse effects are due to the antihistamine, and dyes and excipients used in the formulation may be responsible for urticaria, angioedema and asthma. Syrups contain preservatives, artificial flavours and colouring agents. A number of drugs are now free of these additives and they are to be preferred in treating chronic urticaria.

TABLE 5.5 **Some commonly used antihistamine tablets or capsules which contain no dyes**

• Astemizole	• Cyproheptadine	• Pheniramine
• Azatadine	• Diphenylpyraline	• Terfenadine
• Cetirizine	• Loratadine	• Triprolidine (with pseudoephedrine)

Note: All syrups, elixirs and suspensions contain dyes, preservatives and/or artificial flavours. (Adapted from Aldrich RD, Main RA, Smith ME. Dyes and preservatives in oral antihistamines. *Br J Dermatol* 1980; 102: 545–9).

The future

We now have a wide range of drugs available which are highly effective H1 receptor blockers and which are safe and relatively free of unwanted side effects. Fexofenadine will be introduced soon for clinical use. It is the active metabolite of terfenadine and is free of cardiotoxicity but in other respects is similar to the parent compound. More antihistamines are in the offing, many with other anti-allergy properties. These include ebastine (a second generation non-sedating antihistamine with a profile similar to terfenadine), azelastine (a topically active agent with some anti-leukotriene activity in guinea pigs), mequitazine (a derivative of promethazine which is useful in reducing pruritus), tazifylline (a theophylline piperazine derivative which significantly reduces histamine-induced bronchospasm in experimental animals) and oxatomide (a serotonin and leukotriene antagonist which inhibits histamine release from mast cells and is effective in reducing pruritus). These and other drugs are at various stages of development. Some have been approved for use in overseas countries but are not yet available in Australia, some have not yet been tried in human studies and their places in clinical medicine have yet to be established.

Further reading

Bousquet J, Michel F-B. Are antihistamines really antihistamines? *Allergy and Clinical Immunology News* 1990; 2: 11–15.

Simons FER, Simons KJ. The pharmacology and use of H1-receptor-antagonist drugs. *N Engl J Med* 1994; 330: 1663–70.

Sutherland DC. Antihistamine agents: new options or just more drugs? *Med J Aust* 1989; 151: 158–62.

Chapter 6

Corticosteroids and other drugs

Corticosteroids

Introduction

Corticosteroids are valuable drugs widely used in allergy practice. They are the most convenient and effective anti-inflammatory, anti-allergic and immunosuppressive drugs generally available, but it is well known that their use comes at a price. The manner in which they are used needs to be tailored to the indication, and this discussion will cover their use only in allergic diseases.

Administration

Corticosteroids may be administered systemically by the oral route, or by intravenous injection in the more acute situations. Topical preparations are available for use on skin, in conjunctivae, and by inhalation or by insufflation in the nose. Their two principal applications in allergy are to control acute allergic disease and to maintain effective disease control once it has been achieved.

1. *To control acute allergic disease.* If corticosteroids are indicated they need to be given systemically for asthma and generalised reactions such as anaphylaxis or urticaria and angioedema, but topical agents are usually sufficient for eczema and nasal symptoms. The principles of use are to:
   (a) commence with large doses sufficient to control the disease without the necessity of subsequently increasing the dose;
   (b) start therapy as early as possible. If in doubt, err on the side of giving steroids;
   (c) reduce the dose and/or change to topical therapy as soon as possible.

In acute severe asthma, systemic administration should be used earlier rather than later, especially if the patient has required systemic steroids in the past or is on maximal inhaled therapy including steroids. In this situation inhaled corticosteroids are inadequate. However, in the subacute situation with deterioration over a period of time, inhaled corticosteroids should be increased to their maximal dose. A typical regimen in an adult would

TABLE 6.1 Corticosteroid preparations

	Dosage adult (mg)	Equivalent doses (mg)	Indications and remarks
Intravenous			
Hydrocortisone	100–200 6 hourly	20	Acute asthma, allergic emergencies.
Methylprednisolone	500–1,000 single	4	Acute immunopathic diseases, eg renal SLE, vasculitis.
Dexamethasone	2–6/Kg body weight	0.75	Treatment of shock.
Intramuscular			
Depot-methylprednisolone (Depo-Medrol)		No longer indicated in allergic diseases	
Betamethasone, combined soluble and depot preparation			
Dexamethasone	4–20/day IM (or IV)		Control of acute allergic and inflammatory conditions, treatment of cerebral oedema.
Oral*			
Hydrocortisone	30 daily	20	Used mainly as replacement steroids Short biological half-life (8–12 hours).
Prednisolone	Induction 15–200 daily in divided doses Maintenance: 1–25 daily or second daily	5	Preferred to prednisone because of more reliable bioavailability under certain circumstances, eg impaired liver function. Intermediate biological half-life (12–36 hours).
Prednisone	As for prednisolone	5	Required biotransformation by liver to prednisolone. Similar duration of action.
Dexamethasone	Induction: 0.5–10 daily in divided doses Maintenance: 0.5–1 daily in divided doses	0.75	Potent glucocorticoid, less mineralocorticoid activity, valuable for reducing cerebral oedema. Long biological half-life (36–72 hours).
Betamethasone			Deleted 1995

*Oral dosage is determined by the nature and severity of the clinical conditions for which it is indicated.

be hydrocortisone 200 mg IV 6 hourly for 24 to 48 hours, substituting an equivalent dose of an oral drug and then withdrawing or reducing to previous maintenance dosage over 4 to 5 days. In less acute situations, oral prednisolone may be administered in divided daily doses of 60 to 80 mg for 2 to 3 days, reducing thereafter to withdrawal or maintenance over 4 to 5 days. In general, inhaled corticosteroids should not be relied on for controlling acute asthma.

In anaphylaxis and angioedema with obstruction to airflow, intravenous hydrocortisone is indicated as adjunctive therapy. The primary therapy is adrenaline which acts within minutes. Corticosteroids take some hours for maximal effect, which is too slow for these acute situations. However, they are useful for preventing a later recrudescence of the disease.

Systemic steroids are rarely indicated in other situations. Examples are control of acute eczema, or in extremely severe refractory allergic rhinitis. Oral administration is adequate in these situations. There is no longer any role for use of ACTH or injections of long-acting depot preparations.

2. *For maintenance therapy.* The principles of use are to:
   (a) use topical therapy in preference to systemic therapy wherever possible;
   (b) if systemic therapy is indicated it should be used in the least dosage to control symptoms, and frequent and repeated attempts should be made to reduce the dosage;
   (c) systemic therapy should not be used unless the patient is receiving maximal topical steroids or unless these are contra-indicated;

TABLE 6.2 **Side effects of systemic corticosteroids**

Metabolic effects
    Glucose intolerance and diabetes
    Hypokalaemia
    Fluid retention
    Osteoporosis
    Acute electrolyte and acid-base shifts with large intravenous doses
Avascular necrosis of femoral or humeral head
Hirsutes on face
Acne
Increased appetite, weight gain
Redistribution of fat with truncal obesity
Purple striae
Insomnia
Emotional lability, psychosis
Hypertension
Cataracts
Infections
Allergic reactions to methylprednisolone have been reported

(d) doses should be given in the morning rather than in the evening to reduce the effects on the hypothalamo-pituitary axis;

(e) wherever possible alternate day therapy is preferable to daily therapy, which in turn is preferable to divided daily doses.

Side effects

Toxicity of these drugs is well known. Their incidence and severity can be reduced in many cases by careful and intelligent usage. The patient should be made aware of the risks of this form of treatment and it is mandatory that they should be carefully supervised. Some patients will be able to regulate the dosage in accordance with their requirements, as for example in asthma, but this should always be done with the knowledge and approval of their practitioner.

Topical therapy can give rise to systemic toxicity through absorption when used in high dosages, or to local toxicity. Topical effects include skin atrophy (especially when potent fluorinated steroids are used on the face); bleeding and dryness of nasal mucosa; raised intra-ocular pressure (when used for long periods in the eye) and predisposition to viral keratitis; and with inhaled steroids, a hoarse voice and oro-pharyngeal candidiasis.

Mode of action

Clinical implications of corticosteroid effect

Corticosteroids have many and complex actions on inflammatory and immune pathways. At a clinical level it is important to remember that corticosteroids do not affect the immediate allergic reaction. They do not interfere with the wheal and flare response seen in the skin prick test with allergen, and therefore do not need to be ceased prior to skin testing. They do not block immediate bronchoconstriction following allergen inhalation, but they do prevent the late allergic response. Patients on moderate doses of systemic steroids will often have a neutrophil leucocytosis due to redistribution of leucocytes with mobilisation of the marginated pool. Their ability to mount a fever is compromised, and they may not have myalgic and other symptoms, which make it is easy to miss infections in these patients. Because of the anti-inflammatory and immunosuppressive effects, patients on steroids are at increased risk of infection. Systemic steroids also cause lymphopenia and reduction in eosinophil numbers.

Corticosteroids induce glucose intolerance which at one extreme can result in the rapid onset of diabetes and hyperglycaemic ketoacidosis. Blood glucose levels should be monitored at least twice a week in patients on large systemic doses of steroids, and monitored immediately should they present with thirst, polyuria, dehydration, variability in refraction, and visual disturbances, or any unexplained symptoms. These patients can develop hypertension and blood pressure should be monitored regularly. Hypokalaemia may occur with continued systemic use and electrolytes should be monitored. Patients should be warned about fluid retention and changes in facial appearance. There is a delay in the onset of the moon facies, and it may continue to deteriorate initially despite a reduction in steroid dosage. This may cause distress unless they understand that there is a lag between steroid administration and changes in facial appearance, and that the changes are not permanent.

Patients should be warned to discipline their eating habits because of the increased appetite which steroids produce. Mood swings may occur, with depression or hyperactivity. Patients may have difficulty sleeping, especially if corticosteroids are given in the evening.

Adrenaline

Adrenaline is a life-saving drug in allergic emergencies. It must be given as soon as possible in anaphylaxis where the outcome is directly related to the speed and effectiveness of intervention. It acts rapidly when given by subcutaneous or intramuscular injection. The dose for an adult is 0.5 ml of 1/1,000 adrenaline subcutaneously or intramuscularly. Half the initial dose can be given at the site of a local reaction such as an insect sting, as this will slow absorption by causing vasoconstriction *provided it is not on an extremity such as finger or toe*. The other half should be given at a remote site. The dose may be repeated in 5 minutes if necessary. In a child the dose is 0.1 to 0.2 ml of 1/1,000 adrenaline. Intravenous administration is necessary only in extreme situations where there is circulatory failure. Extreme care should be exercised in its use. It should be administered as a 1/10,000 preparation in 100 ml normal saline. The risk of cardiotoxicity is greatly increased with intravenous administration.

Patients can be trained in self-administration of adrenaline, and provided with ampoules with the necessary syringes, needles and swabs, or with prepacked adrenaline syringes (Min-I-Jet) or auto-injectors (Epi-Pen). The Epi-Pen devices are the easiest to use. The shelf-life of the products is relatively short, in the order of 12 months, and it is most important that it be checked regularly and replaced when necessary. Adrenaline must be stored away from the light and below 30°C.

Adrenaline can also be administered by metered-dose aerosol (Medihaler-Epi), but it is important to realise that the dose for generalised allergic reactions is different from that required for asthma treatment. In an adult, at least 10 puffs must be given one after the other. This can then be repeated in 5 minutes if the response is inadequate. The adrenaline spray does not need to be inhaled as it is absorbed mainly through the oropharyngeal mucosa. It may be particularly effective where there is swelling of the upper airways. The advantage of this formulation is that it is relatively stable and easily administered. It is excellent for children and for patients who work in remote areas where ideal storage conditions are not always available. The inhaler can be kept in the glove box of the car.

Theophylline

Theophylline is a bronchodilator with a low therapeutic index, that is there is little difference between therapeutic and toxic doses. It is a phospho-

FIGURE 6.1 **Relationship between plasma theophylline concentration and onset of therapeutic and toxic effects.**

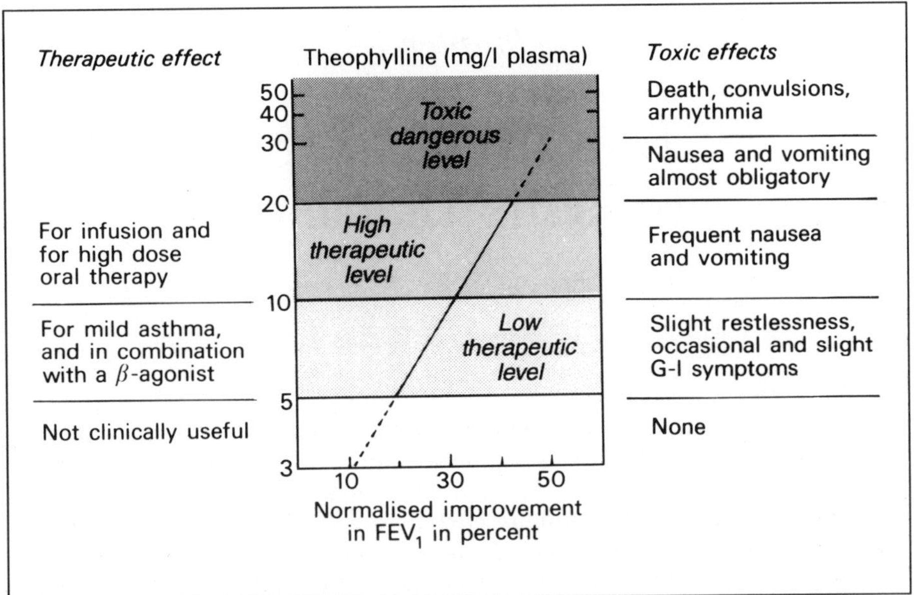

(Reproduced with permission from Mygind N. *Essential Allergy*, Blackwell Scientific Publications, Melbourne, 1986).

diesterase inhibitor, acting by increasing intracellular cyclic AMP levels and leading to smooth muscle relaxation. It is a cardiac and central nervous system stimulant and a diuretic. Nausea and vomiting are frequent side effects, and it can cause flushing, headaches, tachycardia and arrhythmias with palpitations, restlessness and insomnia, and in extreme cases convulsions.

It has gone out of favour in recent times since more effective and safer medications are now available and it adds little to overall management. It is well absorbed from the oral route and long-acting preparations are preferred. Intravenous preparations are available in the form of aminophylline, which is theophylline made soluble by addition of ethylendiamine, and were previously used widely for treatment of acute asthma. However, dosing is critical and must be modified in the light of previous administration of oral theophylline and with cardiac and liver disease. Monitoring of plasma levels is necessary, especially with high dose therapy.

Further reading

Claman HN. Anti-inflammatory effects of corticosteroids. *In:* Clinics in Immunology and Allergy 1984; 4: 317–29.

Chapter 7

Immunotherapy (desensitisation)

Definition

Specific allergen immunotherapy (SIT) is the technique of administering increasing doses of allergens by subcutaneous injection in order to decrease sensitivity to those allergens. Apart from prolonged and profound allergen avoidance it is the only technique currently available which is capable of modifying the allergic reaction. It is also known as desensitisation or hyposensitisation—terms which reflect the clinical effects of the therapy, rather than the process by which it works.

Indications

The conditions for which SIT is indicated are insect sting and respiratory allergies, that is, allergic rhinitis and asthma. Its use in skin allergies such as urticaria and eczema is experimental and it cannot be recommended for normal clinical practice. The same applies to food allergy. Desensitisation, employed in managing certain drug allergies (penicillin, cotrimoxazole), is a different process from that of immunotherapy.

Insect sting allergy. There is no longer any controversy about the value of SIT in management of insect sting allergy. A life-threatening anaphylactic reaction to bee or wasp sting is an absolute indication for immunotherapy.

TABLE 7.1 **Indications for immunotherapy**

Clinical conditions where immunotherapy has been shown to be effective
Anaphylaxis following bee or wasp sting
Allergic rhinitis
Asthma
Allergens which have been shown in controlled clinical trials to be effective
Bee venom
Grass pollen
Ragweed pollen
House dust mite
Alternaria (not commercially available)
Cat dander
Mountain cedar

Lesser reactions, such as diffuse urticaria or increasing local reactions, constitute relative indications, and other considerations need to be taken into account in deciding on therapy, including the patient's age, and access to first aid and resuscitative treatment (see Chapter 18). Sensitisation to the venom must be documented prior to initiating therapy. SIT would not be undertaken in the absence of a positive skin prick test or RAST.

Respiratory allergies. SIT is an accepted form of treatment in allergic rhinitis. However, its use is more controversial in asthma, and opinions have varied from cautious acceptance to outright dismissal. A recent position statement from the Thoracic Society of Australia and New Zealand has supported its use in asthma under strict and careful conditions. Allergic disease which affects several systems strengthens the indication for SIT since it would otherwise require multiple topical therapies.

The following requirements should be fulfilled before embarking on SIT:

1. The patient must have documented sensitisation to a clinically relevant aeroallergen. However, sensitisation alone does not constitute sufficient grounds for treatment. The prescriber must be satisfied that the allergen is a major factor in producing the disease, even though there may also be other precipitants such as cold air, exercise or infections. Prescription on the basis of positive skin tests alone is one reason why this procedure has fallen into disrepute.

2. Symptoms should be sufficiently severe to warrant its use. In allergic rhinitis one would not consider SIT in a disease requiring only intermittent decongestant nasal spray or antihistamines. In asthma there should be the need for regular medication.

3. Exposure to the allergen should be reduced as far as possible. If the allergen can be eliminated completely the need for SIT may be avoided.

   Unfortunately this is usually not possible with common allergens such as house dust mite and pollens.The appropriate course of action for someone allergic to domestic pets is to get rid of the pet, but this cannot always be achieved. The effectiveness of immunotherapy is likely to be compromised by continued exposure to allergen.

4. One or, at the most, two allergens must be identified as being predominantly responsible for the patient's disease. Therapy with multiple allergens has not been shown to be effective and it implies that their individual contribution to the disease may be relatively limited.

5. Patients must be fully informed of the risks of therapy and must have realistic expectations of potential benefits. They should be committed to completing the induction phase without interruption. It may be prudent to defer treatment if travel is contemplated soon after starting therapy.

6. Asthma must be stable, i.e. there should be less than 20% variability in PFR, no nocturnal asthma, medication requirements should be stable and there should be no history of recent acute asthma.

Allergens appropriate for therapy

Only allergens which have been subjected to double-blind controlled trials should be considered for use in everyday clinical practice. Several routes of allergen delivery have been employed in immunotherapy but only subcutaneous injection has been studied in detail and shown to be effective in clinical trials. Sublingual administration is not recommended since adequately controlled studies have failed to show efficacy to date.

Allergen extracts used in Australia for the treatment of inhalant allergy are almost exclusively alum precipitated. These preparations are designed to slow the absorption of allergen, reduce the risk of serious anaphylaxis and provide sustained immune stimulation.

Standardisation of biological activity is a major concern. Mass and concentration of active material is no guide to biological activity. The concentrations of the slow-release preparations available in Australia are expressed in terms of protein nitrogen units and not biological activity. Aqueous preparations of *Dermatophagoides pteronyssinus* which have been standardised against a WHO standard are available. These preparations are extremely potent and their use should be restricted to practitioners who have experience with them.

Prescription of immunotherapy

The decision to prescribe immunotherapy is based on selection of the appropriate patient and antigen, and whether potential benefits outweigh the associated risks. Only a practitioner or team with training and experience in immunotherapy should assume this role.

The principle of therapy is to start with a small dose and gradually increase it as tolerated by the patient in order to achieve a dosage which is effective in immunising the patient. This usually takes about 10 weekly injections. An individual regimen should be tailored for each patient and modified depending on their response. It is the responsibility of the prescribing and supervising clinician to ensure that the doctor administering SIT is comfortable with the procedure, has experience with it and knows when to modify dosage or suspend therapy. He should have access to and be encouraged to remain in contact with the prescribing doctor. He should receive written instructions on patient assessment, precautions and procedures for modifying dosage. It is inappropriate to adhere to a strict dosage scheme. Modifications of dosage may be required during the course of treatment depending on the response. Informed consent according to currently accepted guidelines should be obtained prior to the initiation of SIT.

Administration of immunotherapy

Therapy should be administered only by medical practitioners familiar with the effects of immunotherapy, thoroughly conversant with resuscitative procedures, and in a setting where resuscitative equipment is readily to hand.

Bee venom immunotherapy

There are three possible regimens:

1. *Conventional immunotherapy* consists of weekly injections of increasing doses of vaccine at a rate easily tolerated by the patient. It is the slowest to reach optimal dosage. The patient is at increased risk of an anaphylactic reaction if stung by a bee during the induction phase.
2. *Rush immunotherapy* requires the patient to be admitted to hospital and repeated injections to be given at hourly intervals for 6 or 7 injections. This is repeated once or twice a week until the optimal dose is reached. The risk of a severe reaction is greater with this protocol, but the optimal dosage is reached much sooner and with fewer injections.
3. *Modified rush technique.* The patient is given up to three injections at hourly intervals once or twice a week. Again, the risk of a generalised reaction is greater than with the conventional slow regimen. However, there is evidence that overall efficacy of the rush regimens is superior to conventional immunotherapy.

Respiratory allergies

Pollen immunotherapy should be started outside the pollen season. The risk of adverse reactions is greater if therapy is given during the time of exposure to pollens. There are two regimens of administration thereafter. With pre-seasonal administration, immunotherapy is ceased before the onset of the pollen season. With co-seasonal therapy, injections are continued throughout the year, although there is no increase in dosage during the pollen season, and it may be reduced during this period. With pre-seasonal therapy at least two courses are given in successive years.

House dust mite immunotherapy is started and continued throughout the year. Optimal duration of therapy has not yet been established, but it is customary to continue with monthly maintenance therapy for about three years.

Contra-indications to immunotherapy

1. Severe or poorly controlled asthma is a relative contraindication to SIT. If the FEV1 is less than 70% of predicted, it should not normally be initiated or continued.
2. Unstable asthma, as defined by night wakening, bronchodilator usage greater than three times a week (excluding exercise) and/or peak flow variability greater than 20%, is a relative contraindication to both the initiation and continuation of SIT.
3. The development of bronchospasm or a generalised reaction requires that therapy be suspended and the situation assessed by a specialist to determine whether the risk of continuing is justified. The dosage will require substantial modification.
4. SIT during pregnancy has not been associated with an increased risk of teratogenesis. It should not be started during pregnancy, but there are no specific recommendations about ceasing it should a woman become pregnant.
5. Patients with eczema may notice a flare of their skin disease during SIT

and should be appropriately informed. This may require a reduction in dosage.

6. Although the situation should not arise in patients with asthma, the concomitant administration of betablockers is an absolute contra-indication to SIT. These patients are at increased risk of anaphylaxis and respond poorly to resuscitation.

7. The potential adverse effects of SIT in patients receiving ACE inhibitors is currently under review.

8. SIT for asthma appears to be more beneficial in children than adults, particularly in children with seasonal hay fever and mild co-existent asthma. While no lower age limit has been set for SIT in childhood, most clinicians would not advise it under the age of 7 years.

9. SIT should not be initiated in patients with autoimmune disease or malignancy, although there is no evidence that SIT adversely affects these conditions.

Adverse effects of immunotherapy

Short-term adverse effects are the most important. Local swelling and erythema at the site of the injection is to be expected. It may persist for 24 hours and is not a cause for concern. A reaction over 50 mm in diameter is an indication for reduction in subsequent dose.

Systemic reactions must always be regarded seriously and are an indication for reducing dosage or suspending therapy. They usually occur within 30 minutes of the injection, although reactions may be delayed for several hours with the use of alum precipitated preparations. Generalised reactions include sneezing, bronchospasm and urticaria and in more severe cases, anaphylaxis. Deaths have been reported very rarely, usually in asthmatics, with the use of highly purified soluble extracts and where there was a breakdown in protocol.

No long-term ill effects from SIT have been demonstrated in the many studies so far carried out.

Practical aspects of immunotherapy

Some of the practical issues involved in administration of allergen are the following:

Handling of extracts

1. Extracts should be stored in a refrigerator, clearly marked with the patient's identifier(s) and should be replaced immediately after use. Different formulations of allergen should be stored separately, preferably in different refrigerators. The importance of these precautions cannot be overemphasised since a number of serious misadventures have occurred as a result of failure to identify the correct extract.

2. Extracts should be examined visually for changes in appearance and discarded if necessary. The most concentrated extracts are cloudy due to alum precipitate suspensions, but they should not change colour.

3. The bottle should be shaken well prior to drawing it up to disperse the antigen to avoid variation in dosage.

4. Because most allergen extracts are not biologically standardised, there may be variation between batches. For this reason it is wise to reduce the first dose of a new bottle of extract by 25% to take account of possible variation in biological activity of the preparations.

Patient management

1. Patients should be told to let their doctors know in advance if they are ill or have acute allergic symptoms, in which case the treatment may need to be deferred.

2. Every patient should be assessed clinically on each occasion an injection is given, with particular attention to intercurrent illness, reaction to the last injection, and in the case of asthma, stability of lung function as indicated by peak flow readings.

3. Peak flow meter readings must be taken before injection in every asthmatic patient, and if more than 20% below the optimal value for that patient, the injection should not be given. Peak flow meter readings should be repeated 30 minutes after the injection. A fall of greater than 10% is an indication for reducing the dosage of the next injection.

The injection

1. The medical officer must select and check the correct dose, and must be responsible for administration of the injection.

2. Injections are given subcutaneously, a suitable site being the tissue overlying the triceps muscle group. There should be space to apply a tourniquet proximal to the injection site if necessary. After introducing the needle and before starting the injection, the plunger should be withdrawn to ensure that the needle is not placed intravenously.

3. The patient must remain in the vicinity of the clinic for at least 30 minutes after injection although some centres recommend 45 minutes. The nature and size of the reaction is recorded. Peak flows are repeated 30 minutes after the injection. If there is any fall in peak flow or other untoward effects, the patient is observed for a further period. Thereafter they must not partake of any strenuous physical exercise for the next 6 hours.

Modification of dosage

1. A local swelling larger than 50 mm requires a reduction in dosage for the following injection. With uncomfortable, large local reactions, a rapidly acting antihistamine can be given, and a corticosteroid ointment spread liberally over the site of the injection may reduce the intensity of itching and swelling. Especially with alum precipitated preparations, the onset of the local reaction can be delayed for several hours but anaphylaxis is much less likely with these preparations.

2. Some practitioners 'cover' therapy by giving prophylactic antihistamines

to reduce the local reactions. This may mask a mild reaction and make it difficult to judge the effects of therapy and to modify dosage accordingly. It will not prevent a generalised reaction.

3. During induction if one weekly injection is missed, the following dose should not be increased. If two weekly injections are missed, the following dose should be reduced by 50%. Further delays may require greater modification in dosage. These recommendations may be tempered by particular clinical circumstances, such as previous reactions.

Bee venom immunotherapy

The extracts used are soluble purified venom. The more dilute extracts have a shelf life of only 2 to 4 weeks depending on the concentration. Failure to observe this may result in a severe reaction when a new, more potent extract is used, since the patient would have been receiving a lesser dose than expected. Systemic reactions are more common with insect venom immunotherapy than with alum precipitated preparations. Some systemic reactions are vague, with feelings of anxiety, and it may be difficult to distinguish between anaphylaxis and vasovagal reactions. Serum tryptase estimation is useful in this situation. Levels are raised in allergic reactions.

What to expect from immunotherapy

The success rate of SIT is in the order of 70%—this means symptomatic improvement whereby either no pharmacological agents are needed or their requirements are substantially reduced. For example, they may be needed only at times of heavy allergen exposure. This would still be regarded as successful therapy. Skin prick test results may not change with successful immunotherapy and hence cannot be used as a measure of efficacy.

It is difficult to predict how long therapy will be necessary before improvement occurs. With adequate pre-seasonal treatment of pollenosis, there is usually some improvement with the first season but it is usually much more marked after a second course of injections. With house dust mite immunotherapy, the onset of improvement is variable. It is usually noticeable within 6 to 12 months of initiating injections but occasionally can be later. It is advisable to continue with therapy for at least 12 months before abandoning it.

Bee venom immunotherapy should protect the patient from the general systemic allergic effects of bee sting. This can be demonstrated to the patient by arranging a sting by a bee in the clinic with a drip in place and resuscitation procedures to hand. This procedure is hazardous and should not be undertaken lightly.

Treatment failures

The main reasons for treatment failures with SIT are that the indications were inappropriate or the expectations of the patient were unrealistic. The practice of prescribing SIT on the basis of sensitisation alone (positive skin tests or RASTs) will lead to ineffective treatment. Not all allergens to which a patient is sensitised are responsible for clinical allergic reactions. Inclusion of multiple allergens in a vaccine dilute the relevant allergens to the extent that the immunising dose may be inadequate.

Conclusions

Immunotherapy should be considered a specialised procedure. Used for the correct indications and with careful attention to detail, it is an effective and relatively safe form of therapy. Bee venom immunotherapy offers remarkably effective protection from subsequent stings.

Background to immunotherapy

There are now 60 million patients annually who are treated with specific allergen immunotherapy (SIT) throughout the world. Although not utilised widely in the United Kingdom, this form of treatment has been accepted for many years in Europe and the USA. SIT was first used early this century, and reported by Noon and Freeman in 1911. They considered that pollens were toxins and that by giving regular small doses of the material they were making them more tolerant of their toxic effects. Despite immunotherapy having been in clinical use for over 80 years, it remains a controversial form of therapy. Antagonists charge that the drugs which are currently available are so effective that the risks associated with its use cannot be justified. Efficacy of SIT has been established for insect sting allergy and for respiratory allergies with several allergens.

Cost benefit analysis

An expressed wish by patients to tackle the allergy itself rather than only treat its symptoms, often motivates them to pressure their doctors into considering this form of treatment. The cost-effectiveness of SIT is difficult to quantify. It can be extremely effective in individual patients and is the only approach available currently which offers the promise of modifying the natural history of the disease. SIT should not be regarded as an alternative to effective pharmacotherapy.

In the case of respiratory allergies it needs to be considered in the context of the total cost of asthma in Australia, the mid-estimate of which in 1991 was $652 million (National Asthma Campaign 1992). Asthma medication is undeniably effective and remarkably free of side effects. However, the nature of allergic diseases is such as to require regular medication over many years. Cumulative costs of drugs are substantial. Long-term use of drugs may lead to toxicity, for example growth retardation, calcium, mineral and endocrine effects of high dose inhaled corticosteroids, and possible toxicity of β-2 agonists. Increasingly, the wishes of patients to limit the intake of drugs are being articulated and often form a powerful pressure on the medical profession to find an alternative strategy. Immunotherapy provides an attractive potential for modifying the immune reaction, leading to less need for drugs. Against this must be balanced the cost of the vaccine, the cost of administration, the time involved for the patient, the duration of therapy and the risks involved. A systematic cost-benefit analysis of SIT has not yet been undertaken.

Method of action of immunotherapy

The basic process in immunotherapy is active immunisation, with the expectation that it will alter immune responsiveness to allergen and thereby modify the disease in the recipient. This presupposes that immunological mechanisms play a significant role in the pathogenesis of allergic diseases. The major cellular players in this process are eosinophils, mast cells and basophils, and Th2 cells. There is close interaction between these cells, brokered by release and activity of cytokines with a variety of communication and biological effector properties which attract cells to the site of inflammation and activate them, resulting in destruction of mucosal cells and inflammation. With chronicity of the process, secondary changes occur such as thickening of basement membrane and fibrosis. Modern therapy aims at suppressing the inflammatory process by the use of agents such as inhaled corticosteroid or sodium cromoglycate but these drugs do not have a sustained effect on the inflammatory process and their effects wane after therapy is ceased. Immunotherapy, on the other hand, has the potential for modifying immune mechanisms on a long-term basis.

A number of immunological changes have been described following immunotherapy. These include an initial rise in specific serum IgE, followed later by a fall, and a rise in specific IgG (blocking antibody). Specific IgG titres correlate poorly with the degree of protection in most cases. Immunotherapy leads to reduction in mediator release from mast cells in vitro, and alterations in lymphocyte subsets have also been described. However, its most important function is to deviate T cell function from the Th2 profile which is associated with allergic mechanisms, to the Th1 cytokine profile. This is discussed more fully in Chapter 26.

It could be anticipated that modification of immune events leading to bronchial inflammation would have most effect before irreversible secondary changes such as fibrosis and thickening of bronchial basement membrane have occurred, and therefore there are strong theoretical arguments why SIT should be used early in the course of the disease. SIT may well prove more effective in limiting the progression of chronic cellular infiltration rather than reversing an established inflammatory process. Some data suggest that it may also impact on progression of clinical disease, e.g. its use in rhinitis may prevent the later development of asthma. Definitive scientific data are not yet available to answer these questions.

Evidence for efficacy

Allergic rhinitis

A number of well-conducted placebo controlled trials have shown efficacy for immunotherapy in grass, ragweed and birch pollen allergies. Efficacy has also been established for immunotherapy with house dust mite, but prolonged therapy is required and differences from response to placebo may not appear before a year of therapy. Suitable mould extracts are not available at the present time and SIT is not recommended. One trial with a high quality extract, not available commercially, has shown benefit.

Asthma

There have been 22 randomised placebo controlled double-blind trials of SIT for asthma during the years from 1954 to 1993. Comparison of these trials is difficult, not only because of the inherent problems of trials involving asthma, but also because of difference in allergen extracts and dosage regimens. A meta-analysis can address some of these difficulties and this technique has recently been applied to SIT for asthma (Abramson MJ et al, 1995). The results for changes in symptoms, medication scores and bronchial hyper-responsiveness (BHR) were expressed as odds ratios (OR) for improvement. For SIT with house dust mite, OR for symptomatic improvement were 2.7, reduction in medication 4.2 and reduction in BHR 13.7. For SIT with other allergens (pollens, moulds or animal dander), OR for symptomatic improvement were 4.8 and reduction in BHR 5.5. These odds ratios indicate a clinically useful improvement from the intervention. This meta-analysis concluded that SIT is a treatment option in highly selected patients with allergic asthma.

Bee venom anaphylaxis

Placebo controlled trials with pure venom immunotherapy have shown success in the order of 95% compared with 40% in the placebo groups, which is similar to the results obtained using whole body extract.

Problems associated with immunotherapy

1. *Allergen standardisation.* Standardisation of biological activity is a major concern. Mass and concentration of active material is no guide to biological activity. Concentrations of the slow release preparation available in Australia are expressed in terms of protein nitrogen units and not biological activity. Aqueous preparations of *Dermatophagoides pteronyssinus* are available which have been standardised against a WHO standard. These preparations are extremely potent and their use should be restricted to practitioners familiar with their usege.

2. *Adverse effects.* The report of the Committee on the Safety of Medicines in the United Kingdom in 1986 reported that in the 29 years from 1957 to 1986, there were 26 deaths from immunotherapy, 16 of which occurred in patients where the indication for therapy was asthma. During this period 1,459,273 courses of treatment were administered in the UK. Highly purified and potent aqueous extracts were involved and no deaths were reported with the alum precipitated preparation in use in Australia. Subsequent reports indicated a much lower incidence of anaphylaxis and deaths in France and the USA. One of the major differences in practice between the UK and these countries is that in France and the USA treatment is administered by specialists with expertise in the area. In Australia 5 deaths from immunotherapy were reported to the Adverse Drug Reaction Committee (ADRAC) in the 21 years from 1972 to 1993. Four were asthmatics and in each case there was a divergence from recommended procedure.

Future directions

Although SIT is an old technique, there have been continuing attempts to improve extracts. The ultimate aim is to produce an effective (immunogenic) extract with minimal adverse (allergenic) effects. Chemically modified allergens (allergoids) are not available in Australia but are popular in Europe. These have proven safe and effective. Examples are the adsorption of allergen on to tyrosine as a carrier or treating them with glutaraldehyde.

An exciting new development is the use of recombinant allergen peptides. More and more of the common allergens are now being sequenced so that their amino-acid structure is known, and the important parts of the molecules responsible for inducing the allergic reaction are being identified. These peptides can now be synthesised and are being trialled in diagnosis and in treatment. Recombinant peptides have great potential advantages over conventional allergens for desensitisation because they can immunise patients without the risk of inducing an allergic reaction.

Further reading

Abramson MJ, Puy RM, Weiner JM. Is allergen immunotherapy effective in asthma? A meta-analysis of randomised controlled trials. *Am J Resp Crit Care Med* 1995; 151: 699–74.

Bousquet J, Michel F-B. Specific immunotherapy in asthma.: is it effective? *J Allergy Clin Immunol* 1994; 94: 1–11.

British Society for Allergy and Clinical Immunology (BSACI) Position paper on allergen immunotherapy. *Clin exp Allergy* 1993; 23: Suppl 3.

Committee on Safety of Medicine. CSM Update. Desensitizing vaccines. *Br Med J* 1986; 293: 948.

Current status of allergen immunotherapy. Shortened version of a World Health Organization/International Union of Immunological Societies Working Group Report. *Lancet* 1989; 1: 259–61.

Position paper of European Academy of Allergology and Clinical Immunology. *Eur J Allergy and Clin Immunol* 1993; 48: Suppl 14.

Stewart GE, Lockey RF. Systemic reactions from allergen immunotherapy (editorial). *J Allergy Clin Immunol* 1992; 90: 567–78.

Weiner JM, Walls RS. Specific allergen immunotherapy for asthma. Position paper of Thoracic Society of Australia and New Zealand. *Med J Aust* 1996; in press.

Chapter 8

Prevention of allergic disease

Introduction

When considering measures to prevent allergic disease, one is usually confronted with the situation of preventing the clinical manifestations of disease in an already sensitised individual. This is known as 'late intervention', sometimes termed 'secondary prevention'. The opportunity for preventing sensitisation by early intervention occurs in the infant and is termed 'primary prevention'.

There are two components to the development of allergic disease, namely genetic predisposition, and sensitisation to allergens. Intrinsic genetic factors cannot be altered. However, much can be done to reduce the opportunity for sensitisation by reducing exposure to potential allergens and dealing with environmental factors which predispose to sensitisation. It is important to identify those subjects at highest risk for the development of allergic disease so that they can be targeted. This group offers the best chance of achieving a meaningful effect on the disease process.

Identification of high risk individuals

Atopic subjects are at greatest risk of sensitisation. These individuals respond to environmental allergens by preferential production of IgE antibodies which manifest clinically as allergic diseases such as atopic eczema, asthma and allergic rhinitis. Atopic subjects can be identified by:

1. *Family history.* In infants, the highest risk factor for development of atopy is the family history. The probability of an infant developing allergic

TABLE 8.1 **Principles of allergy prevention**

<table>
<tr><td>

1. *Primary prevention*—to prevent sensitisation
    Identify the high risk individual
    Reduce exposure to allergens—predominantly ingested allergens
    Modify adjuvant factors which encourage sensitisation
2. *Secondary prevention*—to prevent disease in previously sensitised subjects
    Reduce exposure to allergens—allergen avoidance procedures
    Modify adjuvant factors which encourage sensitisation

</td></tr>
</table>

disease if neither parent has allergic disease is 12%; if one parent is allergic, it is 45%; but if both parents have the same allergic disease it rises to 70%. Atopic adults usually give a history of atopic disease in first degree relatives.

2. *The presence of other allergic diseases or a history of infantile eczema or allergic diseases in childhood.* These identify adults at greater risk of allergic disease.

3. *Positive skin prick tests or RASTs to common allergens.* These investigations identify the presence of specific IgE antibodies which are the hallmark of atopic individuals.

4. *Total IgE levels.* Cord blood IgE is a controversial tool for determining the risk of an infant developing allergic disease later in life. It is more reliable when used as a predictive tool in the high risk group with affected parents, than in a random population where its predictive value is low. The rank value of this measurement remains for at least the first year of life, and serum IgE at 9 or 12 months of age may have advantages over cord blood measurements in so far as they are not subject to the effects of intra-uterine maternal factors such as smoking and diet.

Total serum IgE levels in adults tend to be high in atopic individuals, but they do not necessarily correlate with allergic symptoms, and they are not useful for determining which patients are at risk of developing allergic symptoms. In an attempt to increase the specificity of this test, measurement of the aggregate of specific IgE levels has been developed and is available commercially (Phadiatop[R]). This has a role in identifying atopic individuals without determining the identity of the sensitising allergen.

Prevention of allergic sensitisation in infancy ('primary prevention' or early intervention)

Infants appear to go through a vulnerable phase when sensitisation can lead to atopy in later life, and it is therefore particularly important to avoid exposure to allergens in high risk individuals during this period. There is ample evidence that early exposure to protein allergens before the immune system is mature predisposes to the development of allergic disease later. Antigens from ingested foods such as cows' milk, egg and soy can be shown to produce antibodies in all infants, with highest levels of specific IgE in children of atopic parents. Breast milk protects against this reaction. However, antigens derived from the maternal diet can be demonstrated in breast milk in sufficient amounts to cause sensitisation. It is not yet established whether this does in fact occur, although there is no doubt that allergens transmitted in breast milk can induce symptoms in already sensitised infants. On the other hand, there is no evidence that the fetus becomes sensitised to foods in the maternal diet during pregnancy, and modification of the maternal diet during the last trimester has not influenced the prevalence of allergic disease in the infant.

There is good evidence that allergen avoidance in early life reduces the later development of allergic disease. Exclusive breastfeeding significantly reduces the prevalence of cows' milk allergy. The early introduction of solid foods has been shown in some studies to increase the prevalence of eczema in high risk groups, although other studies suggest that delaying its introduction merely delays the onset of eczema. Development of asthma is related more to viral infections in childhood and is not affected by the early introduction of solid foods.

Inhaled allergens can also influence the later development of allergic disease. There is intriguing evidence that children born during the pollinating season for birch trees in Scandinavia have a greater prevalence of respiratory allergies later in life. High levels of exposure to house dust mite also lead to increased risk of asthma and its development at a younger age. The same applies to cat allergens. Holt's work from Western Australia provides a plausible explanation for these observations, in that exposure to inhaled allergens in early life leads to a persistent IgE response, whereas later with maturity of the immune system this response is actively suppressed and a state of tolerance or immune deviation exists.

Allergic sensitisation in infants is facilitated by the presence of adjuvant factors which lead to increased sensitisation to allergens, without themselves inducing an allergic reaction. One of the most important of these is cigarette smoke which increases IgE production. Maternal smoking in pregnancy increases cord blood IgE levels, and smoking in the home can be shown to increase the prevalence of wheezing and asthma in childhood. Bjorksten's

TABLE 8.2 **Primary prevention measures to reduce the risk of allergic disease in the high-risk infant**

1. *Reduce exposure to allergens*
   Breastfeed for at least 6 months
   Possibly restrict mother's diet during lactation, avoiding milk, egg, fish, peanut and soy (value not fully established)
   Avoid supplementary feeding with cows' milk
   No benefit has been shown for soy milk substitutes
   Where necessary, use casein hydrolysate (e.g. Pregestemil, Nutramigen) or elemental formulae (e.g. Neocate) instead of cows' milk or infant milk formulae*
   Delay introduction of solid foods
   Avoid 'allergenic' foods such as egg, cows' milk, chocolate and strawberry for first 9 months
   Avoid pets, especially cats in the cot and bedroom
   House dust mite precautions
2. *Modify adjuvant factors*
   Ensure well-ventilated, dry home
   No cigarette smoking during pregnancy
   No cigarette smoking in the house
   Avoid pollution where possible

*This may be impractical because of cost considerations and some doubt about the degree of benefit which can be expected. Unequivocal recommendations therefore cannot be given at this time. Nutramigen and Pregestimil are available on authority script for the indication of proven intolerance to both cows' milk protein and soy protein formulae under 2 years of age. Neocate has the same restrictions plus intolerance of protein hydrolysate formulae of both whey and casein.

work has shown that pollution and damp homes are also associated with an increased risk of asthma, the latter with an odds ratio of 1.9 which increases to 2.5 if the parents smoke.

Viral infections in childhood are associated with bronchial hyper-responsiveness and can lead to elevated IgE and sensitisation. Trials are currently under way to determine whether this process can be prevented by the administration of long-term low-dose loratidine to susceptible children. The results of this trial are not yet known, and no recommendations can be made. However, young children who develop frequent upper respiratory infection often benefit from an antihistamine if they have excessive secretions with obstruction of upper airways.

The role of alum in inducing allergic disease in humans is still highly speculative. It is widely used as an adjuvant in most childhood immunisations. However, it is a very efficient adjuvant for inducing IgE reactions in experimental animals, and the possibility that its widespread use may be a factor in the epidemic of allergic disease has not yet been seriously examined. It must be emphasised that this possibility provides no justification whatever for withholding immunisations at this time. The risk of non-immunisation far outweighs any theoretical disadvantages of using these preparations in infants.

Some steps, while theoretically possible, are not practical in most cases, such as choosing the month of birth so that it does not coincide with the pollen season. However, some others are relatively easily implemented and are of benefit in high-risk categories. These are outlined in Tables 8.1 and 8.2.

Prevention of sensitisation in the adult

This can be considered as an extension of primary prevention. These measures are worth contemplating in atopic individuals identified to be at high risk of developing allergic disease. Steps which can be taken include:

(a) offering advice in the choice of appropriate work. It is wise for highly atopic individuals to avoid careers which involve significant contact with animals, such as veterinarians and workers with laboratory animals;

(b) selection of appropriate homes if the opportunity arises. Ideally houses should be well ventilated, elevated to allow for ventilation and to prevent dampness and mould, in good repair, especially in relation to gutters and roofs, with smooth floors which are easily cleaned, uncluttered and tidy, and cleaned frequently. If renovations are to be performed where internal walls and ceilings are to be disturbed it is best that the subject move out while work is in progress, since these measures stir up house dust and probably release heavy quantities of house dust mite and other allergens into the environment;

(c) selection of low-allergen plants in the garden. While pollens travel for vast distances on prevailing winds, a local heavy source of allergen pollen can also lead to sensitisation. Advice on the most appropriate plants can be obtained from *The Low Allergen Garden* by DJ Bass, a publication of The Asthma Foundation of NSW (see 'Further reading');

(d) reduction of exposure to rubber or latex gloves by subjects with atopic eczema or with contact dermatitis affecting the hands. This is especially important with health care workers who have heavy exposure to latex and in whom there is a big risk of developing latex allergy.

Prevention of allergic disease in already sensitised individuals ('secondary prevention' or late intervention)

Allergen avoidance should form the primary management procedure in any allergic subject, and it has been shown to be effective in reducing symptomatic disease. Appropriate procedures, as discussed in Chapter 3, include measures to reduce house dust mite populations, to avoid exposure to pollens, to ensure well-constructed, dry houses and limit the amount of rotting vegetation to reduce the growth of moulds. The risk of insect stings can be minimised by a number of simple measures such as the wearing of shoes and socks out of doors.

Further reading

Andrae S, Axelson O, Bjorksten B et al. Symptoms of bronchial hyperreactivity and asthma in relation to environmental factors. *Arch Dis Child* 1988; 63: 473–8.

Bass DJ.The low allergen garden. *Modern Medicine of Australia* 1995; 38: 52–64.

Holt PG, McMenamin C, Nelson D. Primary sensitization to inhalant allergens during infancy. *Pediatr Allergy Immunol* 1990; 1: 3–13.

Norman J. How breast milk protects newborns. *Scientific American* 1995; 273: 58–61.

Stuckey MS. Allergy: its prevalence and the value of early intervention for prevention. *Modern Medicine of Australia* 1994; 37: 121–6.

PART B

Applied Clinical Practice

Chapter 9

Rhinitis

Introduction

There are only four ways in which the nose reacts to noxious stimuli. These
are sneezing, itching, discharge of secretions and obstruction to airflow.
These symptoms are usually present together in variable degree, depending
on the pathology. They may occur in normal people and do not of themselves
constitute a diagnosis of rhinitis unless they are excessive in frequency or
degree and give rise to discomfort.

Definition

Rhinitis is a term which describes inflammation of the mucous membranes of
the nose. Adjacent structures which share the same cell lining are often
inflamed at the same time as rhinitis so that patients may also suffer from
sinusitis, conjunctivitis and obstruction to Eustacean tubes.

Classification

The International Rhinitis Management Working Group published a classification of rhinitis which has now been generally accepted.

Clinical presentation

Allergic rhinitis characteristically presents with sneezing, itching and copious, thin, watery discharge—the so-called 'sneezers and runners'. Nasal
obstruction can be present in allergic rhinitis, especially in the perennial
form due to house dust mite allergy, and sometimes obstructive symptoms
predominate—these patients are the so-called 'blockers'.

Itchy, watery eyes due to allergic conjunctivitis often accompanies
allergic rhinitis, while involvement of the mucous membranes lining the
nasal sinuses and the Eustacean tubes can lead to swelling with obstruction
to drainage of secretions. This can give rise to pain in the frontal and
maxillary regions, to impairment of hearing and to infections of sinuses
and middle ear.

TABLE 9.1 **Classification of rhinitis**

<table>
<tr><td>

Allergic
  Seasonal (hayfever)
  Perennial
Infectious
  Acute Viral infections
    Secondary bacterial infection, e.g. Streptococcus pneumoniae, Haemophilus influenzae,
    Moraxella catarrhalis
  Chronic, e.g. fungal agents, especially Aspergillus species
Other
  Idiopathic (non-allergic or vasomotor rhinitis)
  NARES (non-allergic rhinitis with eosinophilia syndrome)
  Hormonal (pregnancy, puberty, hypothyroidism and acromegaly)
  Drug-induced (e.g. ACE inhibitors, β-blockers, ophthalmic β-blockers, aspirin and non-steroidal anti-inflammatory agents)
  Rhinitis medicamentosa
  Atrophic rhinitis

</td></tr>
</table>

(Adapted from International Rhinitis Management Working Group. *Allergy* 1994; 49 (Suppl 19): 1–34).

Allergic rhinitis may masquerade as continuous or recurrent colds, frequent sore throats, mouth breathing and snoring, a feeling of pressure over the sinuses, recurrent infective sinusitis and headaches. Other atopic diseases are often present, for example atopic eczema or a past history of eczema, conjunctivitis and asthma. Sneezing is usually intense and prolonged. There is intense discomfort from itching of the nose and often intense itching of the soft palate, eyes and ears. The patient uses numerous tissues and handkerchiefs each day because of the copious discharge of thin, clear, watery secretions.

Far from being a trivial complaint, allergic rhinitis can have a significant impact on activities of daily life. Patients often complain of fatigue and malaise, impairment in concentration and headaches. Often the degree of disability is only truly appreciated after they have been treated successfully. These symptoms are explained partly by the discomfort of the disease itself, partly by the treatment, especially if first generation antihistamines or cold remedies are used, and partly by interference with sleep caused by nasal obstruction and post-nasal drip in particular.

Seasonal allergic rhinitis or hayfever is usually due to pollen allergy, most commonly grass pollens which are present in spring and early summer. Symptoms usually start abruptly in spring and may continue for several weeks. The length of the pollen season varies depending on the geographical area (see Chapter 26). In some parts the season is well circumscribed; in other warmer parts there is an extended pollination season, leading to persistent symptoms over many months, often with peaks of intensity corresponding to periods of increased pollens in the atmosphere. Symptoms are usually worse out of doors.

Perennial allergic rhinitis is usually due to dust mite allergy. Symptoms

TABLE 9.2 **Clinical characteristics of allergic and non-allergic rhinitis**

	Allergic rhinitis	Non-allergic/ vasomotor rhinitis	NARES
Sneezing, itching, rhinorrhoea	+++	−	+
Conjunctivitis, lacrimation	+++	−	−
Nasal obstruction	+	+++	++
Other allergic diseases, e.g. asthma, eczema	+++	−	−
Other features of atopy, e.g. family history of allergic disease	+++	−	−
Age of onset	Commonly teens and young adults	Mainly adults and pre-teens	Adults
Nasal mucosa	Translucent, bluish, glistening, enlarged turbinates, may become polypoidal	Dry, pink to red mucosa. Small to slightly enlarged turbinates	
Secretions	Watery, clear, copious	Scant, thick, mucoid	Thin, clear or mucoid

are often severe and tend to be more chronic when the patient continues his exposure to the offending allergen. Nasal turbinates may become chronically enlarged and the dominant symptoms then are obstructive. Other indoor allergens responsible for perennial symptoms include cat dander and cockroach. Cat dander can remain in furnishings and in the internal environment even when the cat is no longer present. One clue may be given by the intermittent symptoms which arise when patients visit homes where cats are present. Mould allergy is also an important cause of perennial symptoms and should be considered when dust mite does not appear to be a major factor. Although perennial, it may account for a peak of symptoms in late summer. Alternaria has been recognised as an important allergen in the drier areas inland to the humid belt of coastal Australia.

The facial appearance of allergic rhinitis is often very characteristic, especially in children (see Figure 9.1). There are dark rings around the eyes, known as allergic shiners, the nose may be swollen, there is a nasal quality to the voice and there is continuous mouth-breathing. The nares may be excoriated from frequent blowing. The face may be elongated from persistent nasal obstruction and mouth-breathing. There may be puffiness of the inferior eyelids. The 'allergic salute' is characteristic where the child rubs the tip of the nose in an upward direction. This tends to relieve the itching and provides a clearer airway. The result is the appearance of a pale crease over the nose about one third of the length from the tip, the so-called allergic crease.

The turbinates in allergic rhinitis are enlarged and have a pale bluish or translucent glistening appearance. With severe prolonged disease polyps

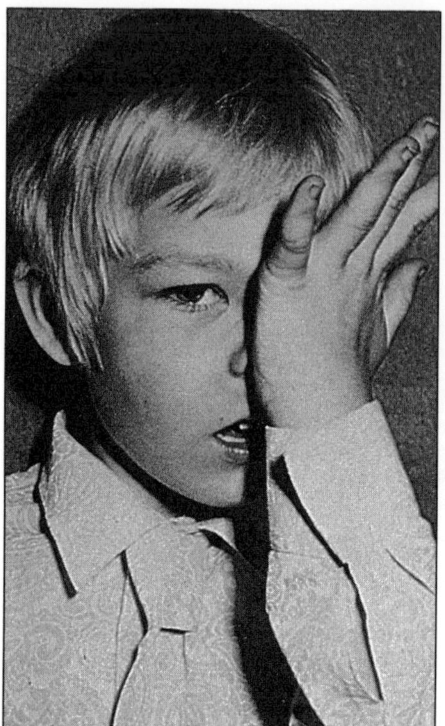

1. The allergic salute.

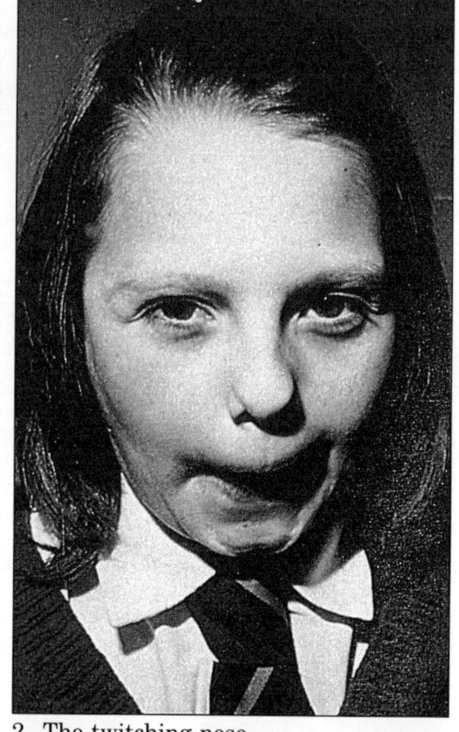

2. The twitching nose.

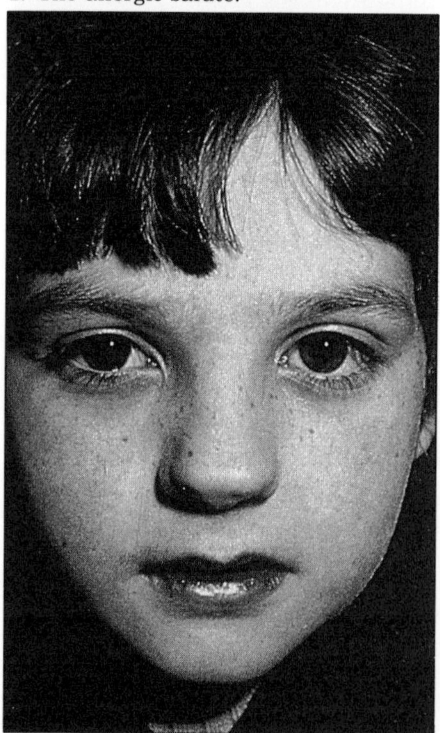

3. The allergic shiner.

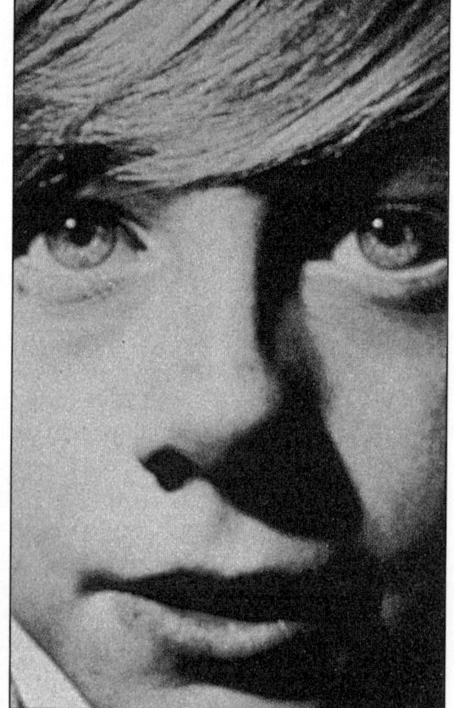

4. Transverse nasal crease.

(Reproduced with permission, Rhone Poulenc Rorer).

may develop. These can be seen as grape-like structures occluding the nasal passages (see Chapter 11).

In non-allergic rhinitis the symptoms tend to be persistent and relentless. Obstruction predominates. Turbinates appear pink or red, dry and of normal size. Patients do not have atopic diseases such as asthma or eczema. There is a subgroup of patients who have episodes of sneezing, watery rhinorrhoea and itching, with marked increase in eosinophils on nasal smears during acute symptomatic periods, and yet no evidence of atopy or any allergic factors. This condition is known as NARES (non-allergic rhinitis with eosinophilia). Its incidence is unknown and its cause is obscure.

Differential diagnosis

Infective rhinitis. The common cold poses great difficulty in diagnosis at the onset of the illness. The initial presentation of allergic rhinitis is frequently that of a persistent or recurrent cold. In both allergic rhinitis and the common cold there is copious watery rhinorrhoea and the patient may feel generally unwell. Patients are afebrile in both cases, although there may be a fever if coryza is an early manifestation of a more severe viral illness. Usually with a common cold the nasal secretions thicken and become discoloured due to secondary infection after 48 hours, whereas watery rhinorrhoea tends to persist in allergic rhinitis. Itching of eyes, nose and soft palate are more prominent in allergic rhinitis. Important clues may be obtained from the history. In allergic rhinitis symptoms have often occurred at similar times in preceding years, or it may be possible to ascribe the onset of symptoms to an environmental factor. The appearance of the nasal mucosa is also helpful. In the common cold the mucosa is reddened whereas in allergic rhinitis it is

TABLE 9.3 **Differential diagnosis of rhinitis**

Infection—common cold
    Prodrome of viral illness (coryza)
Obstructive lesions
    Nasal injuries, deviated septum
    Hypertrophied adenoids
    Nasal polyps
    Foreign bodies
    Tumours
Side effects of drugs including
    Antihypertensives, e.g. methyldopa, prazosin, β-blockers
    Parasympathomimetics, e.g. propantheline previously used in peptic ulcer, more recently for bladder irritability and incontinence
    Topical nasal decongestants
Endocrine conditions
    Pregnancy
    Hypothyroidism
    Menopause
    Menstruation
Cerebrospinal rhinorrhoea

translucent, bluish and glistening. Nasal secretions contain clumps of eosinophils in allergic rhinitis.

Bacterial infection of the nose is rare other than as a secondary event following a viral infection. It is especially important in a child to consider the possibility of a foreign body, in which case the discharge is unilateral, offensive and often bloody. A purulent discharge may also be part of acute sinusitis. The patient may be febrile and has considerable tenderness and pain over the nasal sinuses, and also headache. A rare but lethal cause of nasal swelling, erythema and discharge is mucormycosis, a fungal infection of nasal sinuses which destroys bone. It is confined to poorly controlled insulin-dependent diabetics.

Obstruction due to structural lesions is persistent and often unilateral. In allergic rhinitis it alternates from side to side, and in non-allergic vasomotor rhinitis both nostrils are affected. Tumours are a rare cause of nasal obstruction. They usually occur in adults and are often invasive from or to the pharynx, mouth or orbit. Side effects of drugs and endocrine conditions usually give rise to nasal congestion and obstruction. The antihypertensive agents quoted are not used in modern clinical practice. The same applies to parasympathomimetics such as propantheline which were indicated in earlier years for peptic ulcer disease, but are now used for treatment of bladder irritability and incontinence.

Topical nasal decongestants. Repeated use of drops and sprays containing agents such as pseudo-ephedrine can lead to rebound swelling of nasal mucosa with the need to use even more. Eventually the nasal mucosa becomes dry and atrophic, in its most severe forms giving rise to rhinitis medicamentosa. This is an untreatable, unpleasant condition associated with dryness, discomfort and an unpleasant smell.

Cerebrospinal rhinorrhoea usually results from a defect in the cribriform plate which can result from head injury. It is a persistent, clear, watery, colourless fluid, usually unilateral. Analysis of the fluid will reveal the characteristics of cerebrospinal fluid, that is, the presence of glucose.

Rhinitis in special situations

Infants and children

Classical features of allergic rhinitis are not usually present until after the age of 5 years. However, many infants are snuffly and this may interfere with feeding and contribute to irritability. It is important to determine whether this is infective or allergic. There is a slow increase in incidence of allergic rhinitis to adolescence but most cases of allergic rhinitis start in the teens and twenties. Children often show facial features and mannerisms of allergic rhinitis described above. Chronic nasal obstruction can lead to changes in facial appearance with an apparent lengthening of the face, a high palate, sometimes described as a Gothic palate, and dental malocclusion. Allergic factors should always be considered in young children with recurrent upper respiratory tract and ear infections. Food allergens are often the offending agents in infancy and early childhood. Children rarely suffer from nasal polyps and when they do, it is important to exclude cystic fibrosis and primary ciliary dyskinesia.

The old man's drip and the skier's nose

The conditions under which these problems arise are self-explanatory. They are characterised by watery rhinorrhoea, often profuse. In the case of the skier it is a response to cold. Both conditions respond well to topical ipratropium bromide.

Athletes

Athletes are well represented in the younger age group when allergic conditions are most prevalent, and they are subject to the same problems as patients in general. However, particular care must be taken with therapy on two counts. First, to ensure that medications used are not on the list of doping products. These include vasoconstrictors, systemic corticosteroids and topical corticosteroids, unless accompanied by a physician's declaration. And secondly, to ensure that they do not compromise performance. First generation antihistamines are therefore not suitable for use. Particular care must be taken when prescribing immunotherapy to ensure that they do not train or perform on the day of the injection and that the discomfort of the injection does not interfere with performance.

Investigations

The mildest cases usually do not present to the doctor and these people get by with self-medication or seek assistance from their pharmacists.

More severe or persistent cases merit investigation to identify and deal with reversible precipitating factors. The history and clinical features are fundamental in making a correct diagnosis and in identifying potential allergens and other precipitating factors. *Skin prick testing* should be done in all patients with rhinitis who have sufficient symptoms to warrant a visit to the doctor, with the object of distinguishing allergic from non-allergic rhinitis, and of confirming the identity of potential allergens. RAST is an alternative where skin testing is impractical or contra-indicated.

TABLE 9.4 **Investigations to distinguish allergic from non-allergic rhinitis**

	RHINITIS		
	Allergic	**Vasomotor**	**NARES**
Skin prick tests	Positive	Negative	Negative
RAST (specific serum IgE)	Present	Absent	Absent
Total serum IgE	May be mildly elevated	Normal	Normal
Cytology of nasal secretion	Clumps eosinophils	No cells/basophils	Numerous eosinophils

Total serum IgE may be elevated in allergic rhinitis, but this is frequently not the case and it is an unreliable indicator to distinguish between allergic and non-allergic rhinitis in the individual patient. *Nasal cytology* may be helpful in difficult cases to distinguish allergic rhinitis from infective or non-allergic forms of the disease. In allergic rhinitis there is often an excess of eosinophils which usually appear in clumps. In infective rhinitis there is usually an excess of neutrophils. Peripheral blood eosinophilia is not characteristic of allergic rhinitis.

Nasal provocation with a suspected allergen is a useful procedure for confirming the role of a particular allergen, but this is a specialist procedure and should not be performed on a casual basis.

Radiology. CT scans give much more reliable information than conventional radiographs. They can delineate enlarged turbinates, confirm the presence of polyps and foreign bodies, and may show the presence of a tumour. They may be necessary prior to surgical intervention (see Fig 8.2). Mucosal changes in paranasal sinuses accompany allergic rhinitis in more than 50% of cases and do not of themselves imply the presence of infective sinusitis.

Management

Self-medication and advice from pharmacist

Many patients with mild or intermittent symptoms self-medicate or take advice from pharmacists and may never present to the doctor. The preparations used most commonly include cold and flu preparations, usually a combination of an older, first generation antihistamine with an adrenergic vasoconstrictor drug such as pseudoephedrine. Other patients use nasal sprays or drops containing sympathomimetic vasoconstrictors or antihistamines such as oxymetazoline (Drixine, Sinex, Dimetapp Nasal), methoxamine (Vasylox junior), phenylephrine (Avil, Nyal Decongestant), xylometazoline (Otrivin) or tramazoline (Spray-Tish). With the availability of second generation antihistamines over the counter without a prescription, many pharmacists are now suggesting their use as first line treatment.

Medical management

By the time that patients present to the doctor, they have moderately severe disease and have probably used these medications for some time with only partial relief or with unwanted side effects. The principles of management are the same as for any allergic condition (see Chapter 3). The steps to be taken are as follows:

1. To *identify potential precipitants* and advise on their avoidance.
2. *Topical corticosteroids* are prescribed readily and are very effective drugs in allergic rhinitis. They need to be used regularly as prophylactic agents and are not intended to relieve acute symptoms as they take several days to achieve maximal efficacy. Careful patient education is necessary to ensure correct usage of the drug. Once control of symptoms has been achieved, the dosage should be reduced progressively to the minimum

consistent with control of symptoms. This may sometimes be as little as twice a week. With excessive usage some patients complain of nose bleeds or dryness. These symptoms subside when the drug is stopped or dosage reduced. Continued use of corticosteroid sprays during an upper respiratory infection may prolong the symptoms and it is wise to stop the treatment for a time. Some patients also complain of post-nasal drip of thick mucus with these agents. No ill effects have been described with long-term use of these agents. Preparations available in Australia include beclomethasone (Aldecin and Beconase), budesonide (Rhinocort), flunisolide (Rhinalar), and dexamethasone isonicotinate (in combination with tramazoline as Tobispray). Budesonide is the most potent preparation and is used in a once a day dosage. These agents are not absorbed to any appreciable degree. However, they should be added to the calculation of the total daily dose when asthmatic patients are on maximum amounts of inhaled corticosteroids.

3. *Antihistamines* are often the first line of treatment for patients with allergic rhinitis and other allergic conditions. Antihistamines are best used in anticipation of the onset of symptoms and before exposure to the offending allergen occurs. They are most effective for relieving itching, sneezing and rhinorrhoea, and are less successful in managing nasal obstruction, when combination with an oral decongestant may be more helpful. Antihistamines are particularly useful when multiple organs are involved, such as with the combination of conjunctivitis with rhinitis. The second generation H1 antihistamines are powerful and selective H1 antagonists, and they are devoid for the most part of anticholinergic and other properties. The first generation antihistamines are variably sedating and may interfere with driving, operating machinery or studying. However, they are cheaper than the newer drugs and can be given as a nocturnal dose with a short-acting, non-sedating drug such as terfenadine in the morning, thereby reducing the cost for the patient.

4. *Oral decongestants* are available without prescription. Sympathomimetic agents commonly used are pseudoephedrine or phenylephrine, often in combination with a first generation antihistamine such as (dex)-chlorpheniramine, brompheniramine or triprolidine. In some overseas countries this combination is available with second generation antihistamines such as terfenadine. They are particularly useful for relieving obstruction and nasal congestion in the short term. They also cause reduction in secretions and this may lead to symptoms of dryness. They should be used with caution in hypertension, angina, prostatism and thyrotoxicosis, and they are contra-indicated in patients taking monoamine oxidase inhibitor antidepressants. Side effects include restlessness, insomnia and tachyarrhythmias.

5. *Other topical therapies* include the following:

    (a) *Decongestant nasal sprays or drops* are freely available and widely used. They are useful when starting therapy if there is severe nasal obstruction which prevents access for inhaled corticosteroids. They give prompt but short-term relief of symptoms, especially nasal obstruction. Unfortunately frequent usage results in rebound congestion. Significant tachyphylaxis occurs leading to the use of increasing doses to obtain the required effect. More prolonged and excessive use can lead to rhinitis medicamentosa, an unpleasant condition associated with mucosal atrophy which is refractory to treatment.

(b) *Sodium cromoglycate* is an effective prophylactic drug in allergic rhinitis but needs to be administered frequently, at least four times daily. Its popularity has waned and it has been replaced in large measure by topical corticosteroids. However, it is a safe preparation, free of side effects, apart from transient stinging in a few patients, and is particularly useful in children. The ophthalmic preparation is very effective in allergic conjunctivitis. Unlike its use in other situations where it needs to be used prophylactically, it seems to have an immediate effect in the eye.

(c) *Ipratropium bromide.* This atropine-like anticholinergic agent is very effective in reducing watery rhinorrhoea without being anti-allergic. It gives symptomatic relief in non-allergic rhinitis with severe rhinorrhoea, it prevents the streaming in the common cold and is effective in 'switching off' cold-induced rhinorrhoea such as in 'skier's nose' and in 'old man's drip'.

(d) *Levocabastine* is a topically active antihistamine which is highly effective in relieving both nasal and eye symptoms. It has a rapid onset of action within minutes with duration of action sufficient to allow twice daily dosing. It is well tolerated with a side-effect profile similar to placebo. There is minimal systemic absorption. Patients should not wear soft contact lenses while using this agent. The usual dosages are two sprays in each nostril twice a day, and for the ophthalmic preparation, one drop in each eye twice a day. The dosages may be increased to three or four times a day. Treatment duration should not exceed 8 weeks.

6. *Consider physical measures for symptomatic relief.* Nasal obstruction frequently resolves while the patient exercises and physical fitness seems to have a beneficial effect on allergic diseases. Many subjects derive symptomatic benefit from inhaling menthol, camphor and eucalyptus preparations which have been shown to increase the sensation of airflow through producing a cooling sensation. Nebulised saline and wetting agents such as propylene and polyethylene glycol improve nasal obstruction. Saline sprays are commercially available which offer a simple method of administration. Steaming on a regular basis with the addition of Friar's balsam (benzoin, USP), menthol or eucalyptus is soothing and beneficial where there are thick secretions and obstruction. Mucolytic agents such as benzhexine are also helpful for patients with thick secretions and sinusitis.

7. *Systemic steroids* are indicated for allergic rhinitis in only exceptional circumstances, apart from the treatment of an accompanying generalised severe allergic reaction or in severe asthma. A short course of oral steroids can be useful in very severe disease when there is intense irritability of the nose or severe obstruction unresponsive to therapy and which prevents

TABLE 9.5 **When should a patient be referred to a specialist?**

- If the diagnosis is in doubt
- If the precipitating factor is not identified
- If there is failure to respond to conventional therapy
- If there is interference with normal daily activities or sleep
- If there are complications of the disease, e.g. sinus infection, wheezing
- If there are complications of therapy
- If facilities are not available for performance and interpretation of skin prick tests
- If desensitisation is contemplated

access for inhaled corticosteroids. There is no justification for the use of depot injections of steroids which have been used in the past for seasonal allergic rhinitis now that other effective and more easily controlled medication is available.

8. *Immunotherapy (desensitisation).* This is an effective form of therapy in selected patients. It is the only means currently available which offers the potential to modify the underlying disease process and reduce the reliance on continued drug therapy. It is an adjunct to drug therapy and not an alternative to this form of therapy. It should be prescribed only by those experienced in its use and only after allergen avoidance and drug treatment have been instituted (see Chapter 7 for details).

9. *Surgery.* The usual indication for surgery is persistent nasal obstruction due to anatomical factors such as deviated septum, removal of polyps or occasionally reduction of enlarged turbinates which are refractory to treatment. It may also be required for management of chronic sinusitis. Surgery will often give great short-term benefit. Unfortunately the condition tends to recur unless appropriate steps are undertaken to deal with allergic factors leading to the problem in the first place.

Prognosis

Allergic rhinitis starts most commonly in late childhood and especially in adolescence, and usually improves by middle life. It is unusual for it to be a problem in the elderly, although it has been known to start at any age. Little is known about the factors which determine whether it will go into remission, although common sense suggests that attention to allergen exposure and adequate treatment favour resolution of the problem.

Background

Functions of the nose

Air-conditioner. The primary function of the nose is to act as an air-conditioner for inhaled air before it enters the lungs. It is a highly efficient organ and depends on sophisticated mechanisms to achieve its purpose. This process consists of:

(a) removal of particulate matter. The grid of hairs at the vestibule remove the larger particles, while smaller particles are trapped in mucus which is then removed by ciliary action to the back of the nose;

(b) humidifying the inhaled air to approximately 100%;

(c) conserving exhaled water and heat, a process of great importance in extreme conditions.

Sense of smell. Smell is a primitive sense essential for survival in some species. In man, it determines our sense of taste, well appreciated by those whose nasal air passages are chronically obstructed and who lose their sense of taste as a result. It may still have a subtle social role in humans analogous to the role of pheromones in other species.

Functional anatomy

The nose is a narrow chamber 10 to 12 cm in length. Along the lateral walls are three elongated pads of tissue, the nasal turbinates which fluctuate in size depending on conditions and which function by rendering the airflow turbulent. The openings to the nasal sinuses (ostia) are very narrow and are situated beneath the turbinates. They are easily blocked by mucosal swelling.

FIGURE 9.2 **The lateral wall of the nasal cavity showing the turbinates and the positions of the ostia of the paranasal sinuses.**

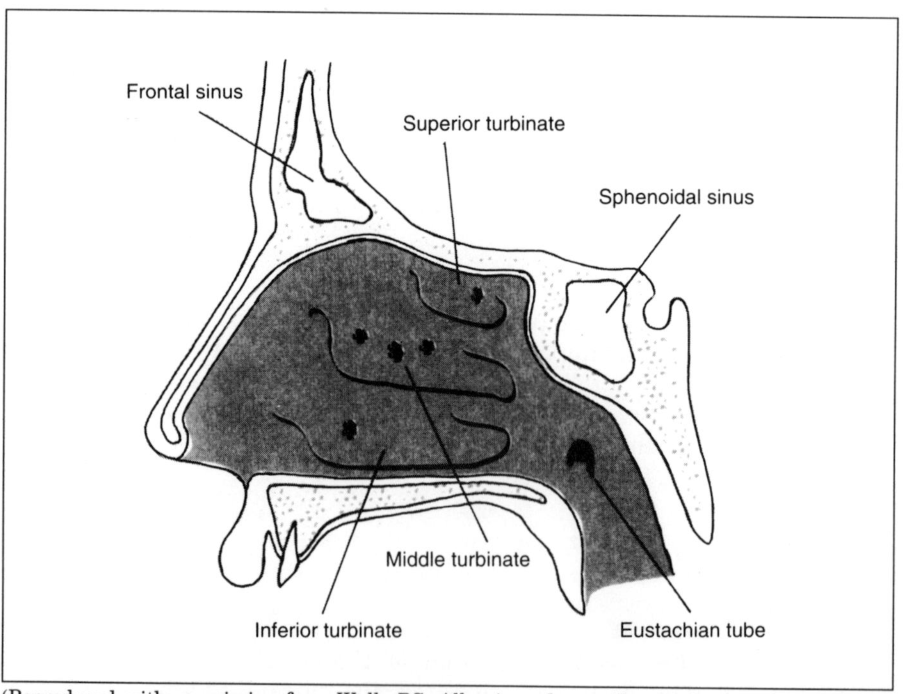

(Reproduced with permission from Walls RS. Allergic and non-allergic rhinitis: diagnosis and management. *Modern Medicine of Australia* 1994).

FIGURE 9.3 Neurovascular connections in the nose.

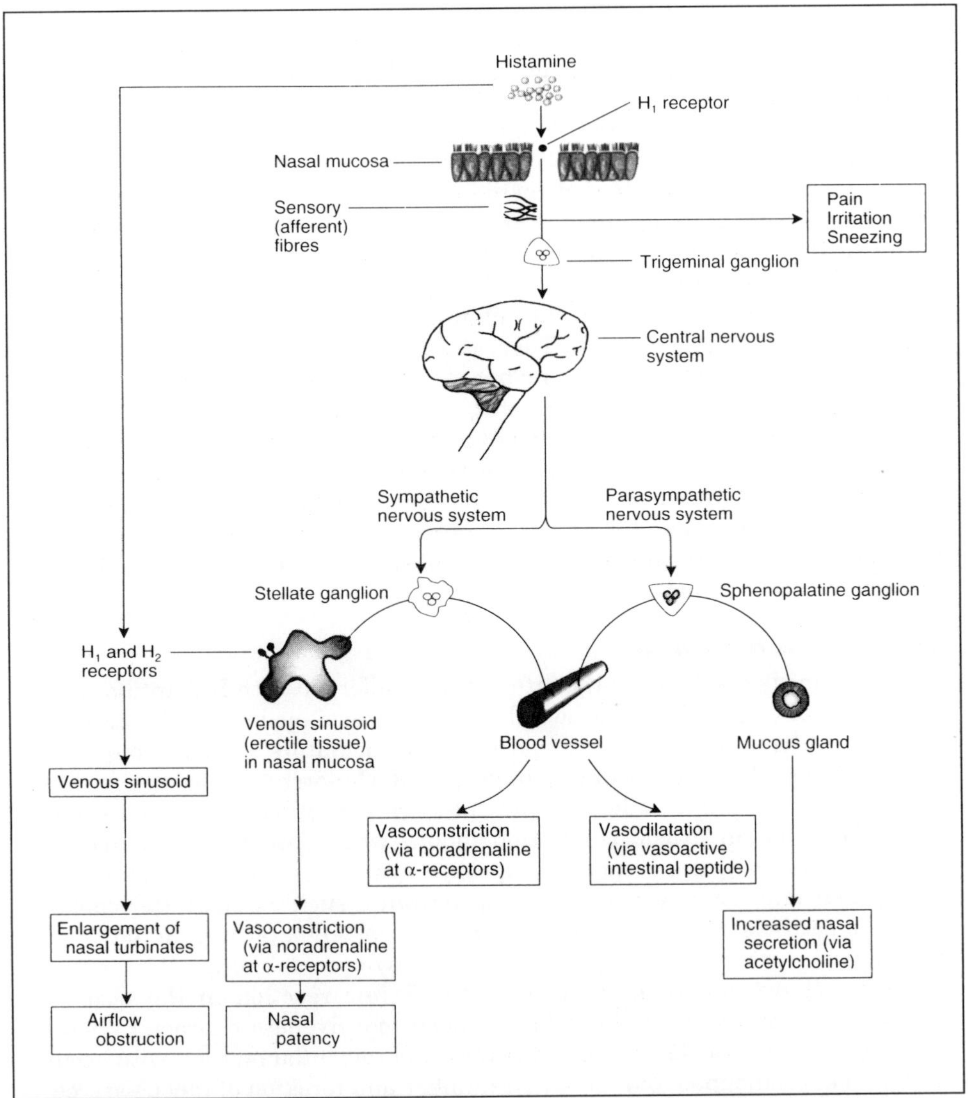

(Reproduced with permission from Walls RS. Allergic and non-allergic rhinitis: diagnosis and management. *Modern Medicine of Australia* 1994).

The ostia to the maxillary sinuses are situated beneath the superior turbinates so that drainage from the sinuses is against gravity.

Secretions. There are large numbers of secretory glands throughout the nasal mucosa responsible for humidifying the air. Secretions are of two kinds—mucus and watery. Large volumes are secreted each day.

Vascular tissue. The nose is a highly vascular organ. Turbinates have abundant venous sinusoids with extensive arteriovenous anastomoses and smooth muscle in their walls which function as erectile tissue, expanding and contracting under neural control.

Nerve supply. The nose is richly supplied with nerves. Sympathetic innervation is through the stellate ganglion, and sympathetic discharge causes vasoconstriction of the venous sinusoids and blood vessels. Parasympathetic innervation derives from the facial nerve via the vidian nerve and the sphenopalatine ganglion. Stimulation results in vasodilatation with consequent venous engorgement and increased nasal secretion via the effect of acetylcholine on mucous glands. Small afferent nerve endings are found throughout the mucosa, many in close proximity to mast cells. Histamine stimulates these nerve endings directly.

Mast cells are numerous in the submucosa, and basophils are present in secretions overlying the mucosa. There is a close relationship between mediator release and neurovascular responses. Histamine stimulates afferent nerve endings directly, leading to sneezing and itching, and initiating reflexes which cause venous engorgement and increased secretion from mucous glands. Histamine causes dilatation of venous sinuses directly through H1 and H2 receptors. Other mast cell and basophil mediators also contribute to symptoms. Leukotrienes C4 and D4 increase mucosal blood flow, increase vascular permeability and induce nasal obstruction. Prostaglandin D2 is extremely potent in increasing nasal airways resistance.

Pathogenesis of rhinitis

Allergic rhinitis results from the interaction of allergen with IgE antibody on the surface of mast cells and basophils with release of mediators. The clinical picture results from the interaction of these mediators with receptors on target tissues. Intense sneezing, itching and rhinorrhoea develop within minutes of instilling an allergen into the nose of a subject allergic to that particular allergen. Nasal congestion follows with obstruction to airflow. With more prolonged or repeated exposure symptoms become chronic and obstruction may become more obvious. Irritants such as cigarette smoke, pressure aerosols and perfumes, and changes in temperature, humidity or barometric pressure may exacerbate symptoms due to nasal hyperresponsiveness induced by the late allergic reaction in the nose, a situation analogous to the bronchial hyperresponsiveness characteristic of asthma. The mucosa shows signs of chronic allergic inflammation with accumulation of eosinophils and increased number and function of mucus-secreting glands.

In non-allergic vasomotor rhinitis, tissues are chronically inflamed and turbinates enlarged. Obstruction is the predominant feature and there is little sneezing or itching.

Further reading

Davies RJ, Ollier S, Cundell DR. Drug treatment for nasal allergy. *Clin exp Allergy* 1989; 19: 559–68.

International Consensus Report on the Diagnosis and Management of Rhinitis. *Allergy* 1994; Suppl 19: 5–34.

Mygind N. Nasal allergy. Melbourne: Blackwell Scientific Publications, 1978.

Chapter 10

Allergy involving the eye

Introduction

The eye is frequently affected by allergy producing allergic conjunctivitis, either alone or as part of allergic rhinitis. More severe, but less common is vernal keratoconjunctivitis. Other parts of the eye may be affected by immunological reactions and eye involvement may occur as part of a generalised disease process.

Allergic conjunctivitis

This is the most common allergic disease of the eye. It is almost invariably associated with allergic rhinitis of some degree which, even if not immediately obvious, will become apparent on examining the nose. Allergic conjunctivitis is usually, but not invariably, bilateral. Unilateral disease may occur from directly instilling an allergen into the eye, for example by a cat-allergic patient rubbing her eye after touching the cat. Itching is the most prominent symptom. This causes the patient to rub the eyes which exacerbates the condition. Conjunctivae are injected in the classical distribution with the emphasis of redness being present peripherally. There may be chemosis (oedema of the conjunctivae) and a clear or opalescent discharge, usually watery, but which may be stringy in severe cases. There may be swelling of the eyelids. The palpebral conjunctivae often appear reddened, dry and granular.

Differential diagnosis

Infective conjunctivitis. Stinging and pain is more obvious than itching; discharge is thick, discoloured and lids stick together in the morning from inspissated pus.

Scleritis and episcleritis. The globe is reddened in a more localised fashion, may bulge from scleromalacia and there is pain which is often deep-seated.

Iritis. Pain is more prominent, and the distribution of injection is different with emphasis around the limbus.

Ocular cicatricial pemphigoid is a disease of older people with prominent shortening of the limbic conjunctiva and loss of the conjunctival sac due to scarring contractures.

Investigations

The clinical picture is usually characteristic. However, if in doubt, corneal secretions can be smeared on a glass slide and examined for eosinophils.

Responsible allergens need to be identified from the history supported by skin prick testing.

Management

General principles of management of allergic diseases apply, i.e. identify and remove potential allergens, reduce the symptoms, inhibit the allergic reaction and consider immunotherapy.

Decongestant and antihistamine eye drops give quick but temporary relief after an initial stinging in some cases. A new potent topical antihistamine preparation, levocabastine, is now available for use in eyes and as a nasal spray. The dose is one drop in each eye twice a day. Care should be taken to ensure that eye drops remain sterile and are discarded as indicated on the package.

Sodium cromoglycate 2% gives immediate and effective relief of symptoms and in this respect is unlike the same preparation used in the lungs or nose where efficacy builds up over weeks. Sodium cromoglycate is intended to be used as a prophylactic agent every 4 to 6 hours, as it is in the nose and lung, but in the eye it appears to be effective also when used on an as required basis. Vernal conjunctivitis is the approved indication for authority prescription but it works very well in allergic conjunctivitis.

Corticosteroid eye drops give effective relief when other measures fail. However, their use is associated with unwanted side effects when continued for a prolonged period. These include viral keratitis and increased intraocular pressure with onset of open angle glaucoma.

Vernal conjunctivitis (keratoconjunctivitis)

This is a relatively rare, chronic and severe condition which occurs in spring and summer, although allergens cannot usually be incriminated. It tends to occur in warm climates, affects young people and males predominantly, and it usually undergoes resolution in 5 to 10 years. The aetiology is unknown. However, it has features of atopic disease, with a family history of atopy in 75% of cases, positive skin tests and raised serum IgE, and pathological changes characteristic of allergy with the presence of mast cells, eosinophils, and elevated histamine levels in ocular discharge. Unfortunately the offending allergen or allergens are seldom identified.

Conjunctivae show a characteristic cobblestone appearance produced by the presence of large nodules in palpebral conjunctivae. Secretions are stringy. There is intense irritation with itching, an intense desire to rub the eyes, redness and photophobia, and keratitis occurs frequently.

Differential diagnosis includes trachoma in some regions. Giant papillary conjunctivitis can occur in association with the use of contact lenses.

Management. It does not respond to topical antihistamines and decongestants. In acute exacerbations topical corticosteroids need to be used. Sodium cromoglycate should be used prophylactically 4 to 6 times a day, especially during the spring and summer season, as it may reduce the total dose of steroids necessary. Antibiotics are indicated for secondary infection, sometimes superficial keratectomy is required for a mucous plaque on the cornea, and a mucolytic agent such as 10–20% solution of acetylcysteine may be helpful when there is a copious thick mucous discharge.

Diseases affecting eyelids

The eyelids may be affected by contact dermatitis, usually from cosmetics, and by severe atopic eczema. Eyelids are also affected by angioedema as the tissues are soft and readily accumulate fluid. Topical steroids can be applied as for the face, avoiding the more potent fluorinated preparations and using only hydrocortisone, mometasone or methylprednisolone aceponate. Care must be taken to avoid eye contact with the ointment and sometimes ocular corticosteroid preparations need to be used at the same time.

Other structures of the eye

Allergic (IgE mediated) conditions do not usually affect other structures of the eye, although they are vulnerable to immunopathic processes, either alone or as part of a general medical condition. The lens may be affected by prolonged steroid administration with the premature development of cataracts.

Further reading

Friedlaender MH. Ocular allergy. *In:* Allergy Principles and Practice. 4th Ed. Middleton Jnr E, Reed CE, Ellis EF, Adkinson Jr NF, Yunginger JW, Busse WW (eds). St Louis, USA: Mosby, 1993; 1649–60.

Chapter 11

Disease of upper airways and related structures

Nasal polyps

Nasal polyps are oedematous extensions of mucous membrane arising from ethmoid and other paranasal sinuses by a stalk. They have the structure of the nasal mucosa and are filled with oedema fluid.

Classification

Non-allergic polyps. More than half of polyps arise in patients without rhinitis or with non-allergic rhinitis. It has been suggested that chronic infection may play a role in their formation. Certainly their presence predisposes to infection.

Allergic polyps. Long-standing, severe and untreated allergic rhinitis can result in polyp formation.

Association with cystic fibrosis. Most polyps in children are associated with cystic fibrosis, so that a sweat test becomes a mandatory investigation in these circumstances.

Nasal polyposis, aspirin hypersensitivity and intrinsic (late onset) steroid-dependent asthma (Samter's triad). These patients have recurrent multiple nasal polypi and at some stage of their illness develop severe hypersensitivity to aspirin with the development of an anaphylactoid reaction to aspirin and NSAIDs. Asthma is usually moderately severe and steroid-dependent. The three components of the triad may develop sequentially and in any order.

Clinical features

Polyps give rise to symptoms of obstruction, and a sensation of fullness or pressure in the nose and of wanting to clear the nose by blowing but of being unable to. By interfering with drainage, polyps predispose to recurrent sinus infections. Post-nasal drip is another troublesome symptom. There is characteristically a disabling loss of sense of smell and consequent loss of sense of taste. Polyps may be asymptomatic but they tend to progress slowly over many years.They are often recurrent and removal is followed some months later by further polyps and a return of symptoms.

Investigations

Allergy investigations may be required to exclude allergic rhinitis. Radiology of the nose and nasal sinuses is necessary to establish the extent of involvement.

Differential diagnosis

Particularly when obstruction is limited to one side, the possibility of other space-occupying lesions needs to be considered, including tumours.

Management

Usually polyps respond poorly to medical management, including the topical application of vasoconstrictors and steroids, and surgical removal is required. It is important to identify allergic factors since their persistence leads to recurrence after surgical removal. Aggressive treatment for allergy, including allergen avoidance, topical corticosteroids, antihistamines and where indicated immunotherapy may prevent recurrence of polyps. Associated infection should be managed appropriately. Postoperatively the recurrence of polyps can be delayed by regular use of intranasal steroids, and this is particularly indicated with a history of multiple polypectomies.

Sinusitis

Definition

Many patients complain of chronic sinusitis (or 'sinus') when they mean perennial rhinitis. The strict meaning of the term 'sinusitis' is inflammation of paranasal sinuses usually caused by infection. It may be acute or chronic/recurrent. About 40% of atopic patients with allergic rhinitis and/or asthma have radiological evidence of involvement of sinuses but with no evidence of infection. There are more goblet cells in sinuses so that secretions tend to be thicker and stickier than nasal secretions.

Clinical features

Patients present with pain over cheeks, forehead, or behind the eyes or with a feeling of fullness in the head. The pain can be intense, especially with changes of pressure such as are experienced with flying. There may be a purulent discharge, often post-nasally. The patient may have a nasal voice, a flush over maxillae and tenderness to palpation over the sinuses. Mucopurulent discharge is present in the nose, the mucosa appears red and inflamed and polyps may be visible with the nasal speculum. A useful indication that sinusitis has developed is the change in cytology of nasal secretions from eosinophils to neutrophils.

Differential diagnosis

Nasal obstruction occurs in allergic and non-allergic rhinitis and there may be radiological evidence of sinus mucosal involvement without infection.

Dental problems of the upper jaw such as root abscess can give rise to pain similar to that of sinusitis. Nasal polyps give rise to similar symptoms in the absence of infection, although they predispose to infection by causing nasal obstruction. Tumours of the paranasal sinuses are rare. Fungal infections may be invasive and lethal. Mucormycosis occurs in uncontrolled diabetes mellitus and carries a high mortality.

Immunodeficiency states can present with recurrent sino-pulmonary infections, and this possibility should always be considered in patients who have recurrent infections, especially if the infections involve the lungs and also occur in other sites. These conditions are rare but important to diagnose since early treatment will prevent the onset of irreversible changes.

Investigations

Evidence of mucosal thickening of greater than 5 mm and polyps or fluid levels on CT scan indicate mucosal involvement, but this does not necessarily indicate that infection is present. The same picture can arise with allergic rhinitis.

Management

Antibiotics are indicated for acute infection and for acute exacerbations of chronic sinusitis. The most common organisms are Streptococcus pneumoniae, Haemophilus influenzae and Moxarella catarrhalis, although anaerobic organisms are also frequent offenders. The antibiotics of choice are amoxycillin or roxithromycin.

With recurrent or chronic sinusitis, full assessment should be undertaken to exclude nasal polyps in adults and other mechanical factors that can interfere with drainage. A full diagnostic work-up should be undertaken for allergic factors which predispose to sinusitis by causing oedema of nasal mucosal tissues.

Allergy affecting the ear

Contact and atopic eczema

The pinna and external auditory meatus can be affected by atopic eczema with scaling and cracking. Contact eczema is commonly due to earrings, especially 'silver' ones which have a high nickel content.

Serous otitis media

Serous otitis media, also known as glue-ear, usually affects children and is a common cause of deafness in this age group. The middle ear is normally air-filled with only a minimal amount of fluid. Cells lining the cavity are cuboidal, but goblet cells are present. The aetiology is unknown and the role of allergy is controversial. One suggestion is that with chronic obstruction to the Eustacean tube there is failure to equalise pressures in the middle ear with the environment. This leads to negative intra-aural pressure, resulting in hypertrophy of goblet cells with excessive secretion of fluid. Secretions are initially mucoid but as the disease advances they become increasingly viscid and deeper in colour. They interfere with the normal functioning of the bones of the middle ear, finally immobilising them and causing complete deafness. There is no indication of bacterial infection, but it may predispose to secondary infection.

Allergic factors can contribute to the disease by causing chronic obstruction to the Eustacean tube. Many patients have allergic rhinitis and features of atopy. The tissues of the middle ear itself cannot respond to allergic influences. The role of food allergy is controversial. There is a belief that milk can lead to increased viscosity of secretions, although there is little evidence to support this.

The primary management is mechanical and drainage may be required by insertion of grommets. However, a survey to exclude reversible allergic factors is worthwhile since attention to these factors may restore patency of the Eustacean tubes and allow drainage of the middle ear. Antihistamines and topical corticosteroids reduce mucosal swelling and the use of intranasal saline or steam inhalations, or mucolytic agents may provide additional benefit.

Other upper respiratory syndromes

Recurrent sore throats and pharyngitis

Patients are sometimes referred to exclude allergic factors as causes of recurrent sore throats. It is unusual to find allergic factors in the absence of classical allergic symptoms such as sneezing, rhinorrhoea or a history of asthma. On the other hand some patients with severe, poorly controlled allergic rhinitis will have recurrent sore throats from mouth breathing because of nasal obstruction, and from persistent post-nasal drip. These patients often have prominent lymphoid nodules and stringy mucus on their posterior pharyngeal wall. Rhinoscopy and laryngoscopy may show nodularity in the pyriform fossa.

Post-nasal drip

This is a disabling and unpleasant symptom and can have serious consequences. It is most troublesome at night and interferes with sleep, leading to tiredness and depression. It is likely to arise where obstruction is a prominent feature such as occurs in chronic perennial rhinitis and with nasal polyps. Continued use of nasal steroids and vasoconstrictors can lead to inspissation of secretions and aggravate the situation.

Management. Many patients find some relief if they sleep in a semi-upright position. Nasal airways should be rendered as patent as possible and allergic disease should be treated adequately. Some patients find significant benefit from measures aimed at reducing the viscosity of secretions such as by the use of saline sprays and regular steam inhalations. Sometimes a mucolytic agent such as bromhexine can assist. If polyps are present they may need to be removed.

Persistent cough

There are many causes of a chronic cough with the reflex originating in the lungs, upper airways or outside the respiratory tract. Once causes such as chronic bronchitis, bronchiectasis and bronchogenic carcinoma have been excluded, there remain a group of patients in whom no obvious cause can be found. The question is sometimes raised as to whether allergic factors are responsible for the persistent cough. In some years a number of patients present around the same time and cite a previous respiratory infection as the time when symptoms first appeared, suggesting that some viral infections may be prone to trigger a chronic persistent cough.

It is unusual to find an allergic cause for this symptom in the absence of other allergic manifestations, and many patients are not atopic. However, the possibility of asthma should be considered, especially with a dry nocturnal cough and particularly if the patient is a child. Cardiac failure is another cause of a nocturnal cough which may be overlooked. If other less obvious causes are found (Table 11.1), they should be managed appropriately, for example by ceasing ACE inhibitors, or dealing with gastro-oesophageal reflux by giving ranitidine or omeprazole.

TABLE 11.1 **Some causes of chronic persistent cough**

- Asthma
- Cardiac failure
- ACE inhibitor therapy
- Post-nasal drip
- Gastro-oesophageal reflux disease (GERD)
- Inhaled foreign body (in children)
- Hypersensitivity pneumonitis
- Infections, e.g. M. tuberculosis, H. pertussis, Pneumocystis carinii
- Post infectious, e.g. viral upper respiratory infection
- Carcinoma of lung
- Cystic fibrosis
- Diseases of larynx and pyriform fossa
- Sarcoidosis
- Psychological

If no cause can be found, some patients will respond to a cough suppressant together with some measures to soothe the pharynx such as lozenges or steam inhalations at night. In more refractory cases a trial of nedocromil sodium or ipratropium bromide by inhalation for several weeks will suppress the symptoms. An explanation of the mechanisms involved should be given to the patient together with reassurance that no sinister cause for the cough has been found. They should be encouraged to try to suppress the cough voluntarily.

Further reading

Irwin RS, Curley FJ, French CL. Chronic cough. The spectrum and frequency of causes, key components of the diagnostic evaluation and outcome of specific therapy. *Am Rev Respir Dis* 1990; 141: 640–7.

Lund VJ. Diagnosis and treatment of nasal polyps. *Br Med J* 1995; 311: 1411–14.

Sinusitis

Goodman GM, Slavin RG. Medical management in adults. *In:* Virant FS (ed). Chronic Sinus Disease. Immunology and Allergy Clinics of North America, 1994; 14: 69–87.

Shapiro GG, Virant FS. Medical management in children. *In:* Virant FS (ed). Chronic Sinus Disease. Immunology and Allergy Clinics of North America, 1994; 14: 47–68.

Chapter 12

Asthma

Asthma is showing a true increase in prevalence, particularly in the English-speaking world. It carries a high socio-economic cost for the community since it affects younger people, and has significant morbidity and mortality.

Definition

Asthma is difficult to define in such a way as to embrace all the features and variations of this disease. The result is that there are numerous definitions based on clinical or physiological features. Any definition needs to include the following characteristics:

1. Obstruction to airflow, variable over time, and which is reversible to a degree, either spontaneously or with therapy.
2. Irritability of airways which manifest as excessive responses to a variety of stimuli such as exercise, changes in temperature, irritants and inhalation of hypertonic saline. Bronchial hyperresponsiveness is characteristic of asthma.
3. Characteristic inflammation of bronchial mucosa and submucosa with prominent eosinophils, and desquamation of mucosal cells.

The definition of the National Asthma Campaign includes these features and is simple: 'Asthma is a disease involving airway inflammation. It is characterised by airway hyperresponsiveness and attacks of reversible airway obstruction'.

Classification

Asthma can be classified in a variety of ways depending on the characteristics of the disease which are pertinent to the context. The individual patient may be characterised in several ways which can be useful in defining prognosis, establishing the possibility that identifiable allergic factors may be operating and administering the most appropriate therapy.

Asthma can be classified as follows.

1. Patterns of disease behaviour

(a) *Stable vs unstable asthma.* In stable asthma the response to therapy is predictable, whereas unstable asthma is characterised by marked variability in airflow measurements over time and less than anticipated response to medications.

(b) *Episodic vs persistent asthma.* In episodic asthma symptoms occur intermittently, less frequently than weekly, with normality between. In persistent asthma symptoms are present on a daily basis.

(c) *Perennial vs seasonal asthma.* Perennial asthma occurs throughout the year, while seasonal asthma coincides with environmental factors such as pollination of grass (spring), ragweed (autumn, especially in North America) or trees (birch trees in early spring in Canberra).

(d) *Steroid-dependent asthma.* Determined by the requirement for corticosteroids. Steroid resistance is a special situation (see below).

2. Severity of disease

Criteria for determining severity include requirements for oral or parenteral corticosteroids; admission to hospital in the past for treatment of asthma; dyspnoea at rest; adverse physiological measurements such as hypoxia and hypercarbia; excessive use of bronchodilators, and unstable asthma.

3. Pathogenesis

Extrinsic or atopic asthma occurs in atopic patients with evidence of other allergic diseases such as allergic rhinitis and eczema, and with indications of sensitisation to environmental allergens. *Intrinsic asthma* occurs in the absence of atopy. The onset of asthma in these patients is usually later in life, they have no other allergic diseases, no signs of sensitisation to allergens and no family history of allergy.

The problem with this classification is that it carries the notion that allergic factors are not operating in intrinsic asthma, thus making it unnecessary to look for them. This is a dangerous assumption. Patients may develop sensitisation to allergens at any time of life, and the absence of atopic

TABLE 12.1 **Criteria for severity of asthma**

	Mild	**Moderate**	**Severe**
	Episodic	Persistent	Persistent
Chest tightness	<Weekly	>Once per week	Most days wheezing
Wakening at night from asthma	No	Occasional	>Once per week
Bronchodilator use	<Weekly	>Once per week	Daily
Minimum PEFR on waking, as % of best over 10 days	>85%	70 to 85%	<70%

features or an onset in middle or later life, does not negate the necessity for seeking reversible allergic factors. In extrinsic asthma by contrast, there is often sensitisation to a number of allergens, but none may stand out as being predominantly responsible for precipitating the symptoms.

4. Special categories of asthma

Aspirin-induced asthma is usually severe, steroid-dependent and associated with hypersensitivity to aspirin which can induce a severe syncopal collapse and severe asthma. It may be associated with nasal polyposis when it is known as Samter's triad (late onset asthma, aspirin hypersensitivity and nasal polyposis). Patients with aspirin hypersensitivity also react adversely to non-steroidal anti-inflammatory agents. Paracetamol is normally a safe substitute.

Occupational asthma. The diagnosis is often difficult to establish. Neither the presence of atopy nor cigarette smoking necessarily predict which workers will develop disease.

Exercise-induced asthma. Bronchospasm may be precipitated by exercise in any form of asthma, and the majority of asthmatics have symptoms following vigorous exercise. However, it may be the predominant or only feature in some asthmatics. It is important to recognise as it may indicate inadequate treatment. It is more likely to occur with inhalation of cold dry air, and with jogging rather than with swimming.

TABLE 12.2 **Risk factors for asthma**

<table>
<tr><td>

• Sensitisation to:
   House dust mite
   Cats
   Alternaria
• Family history of asthma
• Cigarette smoke in infancy
• High allergen load in infancy

</td></tr>
</table>

Risk factors for asthma

Genetic factors play an important role in determining the presence of atopy and the risk of developing asthma. Atopy is the strongest risk factor for asthma. Allergy can not only precipitate acute attacks of asthma, but it can also initiate bronchial airway inflammation which is the basic pathological mechanism in this disease. Most asthmatics have some elements of allergic disease. Sensitisation to house dust mite and to alternaria have been shown to be risk factors for asthma. Grass pollen sensitisation, on the other hand, leads to allergic rhinitis but does not appear to be associated with an increased risk of asthma. High levels of allergen exposure early in life lead to increased risk of asthma later in life.

Cigarette smoking in the homes of high-risk infants predisposes to the development of atopy and hence is a risk factor for asthma.

TABLE 12.3 **Evidence for the role of allergy in asthma**

1. Atopy is a risk factor for asthma.
2. Allergy to environmental allergens is a risk factor for asthma
     House dust mite
     Alternaria.
3. There is a statistical correlation between serum IgE levels and the prevalence of asthma.
4. Increased exposure to allergens early in life leads to a greater prevalence of asthma later.
5. Removal of allergen from the environment will lead to a reduction of bronchial hyperresponsiveness over several months.
6. Immunotherapy can be shown to reduce bronchial hyperresponsiveness as indicated by increased histamine PD_{20}.

Triggers for bronchospasm

Viral infections are the most common causes of acute exacerbations of asthma in young children, but they are less important in adults. Respiratory syncytial virus is especially likely to be involved, but adenoviruses have also been implicated to a lesser degree. Bacterial infection is less likely to precipitate wheezing.

Air quality. There is increasing evidence that an increase in particulate matter may be an important precipitant, and this may be one explanation for the worsening of allergy seen with winds blowing from the dry interior.

Allergens such as cat dander or house dust mite precipitate acute asthma in sensitised subjects.

Adverse reactions to foods can be responsible either through allergic mechanisms or through intolerance, and should be suspected when there are sudden and severe episodes of deterioration in asthma. One of the better studied examples is the bronchospasm induced by sulphites where release of sulphur dioxide from food during chewing and swallowing leads to inhalation of the gas which triggers acute bronchospasm.

Other precipitants include cold air, exercise, laughter and psychological stress. These factors operate because of the underlying bronchial hyper-responsiveness which is a hallmark of the condition. Hence non-allergic factors may precipitate attacks even in patients who have allergic asthma and where a specific allergen has been identified.

Clinical features of asthma

In childhood

Cough is a common presentation, especially nocturnal cough which persists despite cough suppressants and which often starts as soon as the child goes to bed. Another common presentation is wheezing in association with viral infections, sometimes called wheezy bronchitis. There is debate as to whether this represents true asthma. Less than one third of infants who wheeze in the first 18 months of life have asthma at the age of 6 years, and it is important

TABLE 12.4 **Triggers for bronchospasm in asthma**

Allergens
  Inhalants
  Ingestants
Infections, especially viral infections in young children
Physical factors
  Exercise, especially jogging, running (swimming is usually devoid of this effect)
  Cold air
  Laughter
Industrial pollutants as inhaled irritants
  Nitric oxides
  Sulphur dioxide
Ingestants
  Sulphites
  Colouring agents, e.g. erythrosine
  Preservatives and additives
  Food allergens
Drugs
  β-blockers
Hyperventilation
Psychological stimuli
Occupational agents

not to overdiagnose asthma in these infants. The airways of children under the age of 5 are relatively narrow and have less elastic recoil than older subjects, rendering them more liable to bronchial obstruction.

In children with chronic asthma there may be deformity of the chest wall with Harrison's sulcus or pigeon chest. There may be evidence of stunted growth due to severe uncontrolled disease, or to the chronic use of systemic steroids, or sufficiently large doses of inhaled drug to be associated with significant systemic absorption. Growth rates appear to be slower in asthmatics, partly as a result of corticosteroids used in treatment, but also from the disease itself. However, in most cases the slowing of growth does not result in any reduction in the final predicted height.

Gastro-oesophageal reflux (acronyms GOR or GER(D) for gastro-oesophageal reflux disease) is common in infancy, but its role in asthma remains controversial. Specialised gastrointestinal investigation may be required in some patients to determine its exact role in precipitating symptoms.

Asthma is an important cause of absenteeism in schools, and particular care may be required in the individual child to ensure that there is an understanding of and sympathy for the condition and to ensure that medications are administered appropriately at school.

In adolescence

Adolescents frequently deny their symptoms and compliance with medication may be a problem. This can lead to an underestimate of the severity of asthma and inadequate treatment with the development of serious consequences.

In adults

Asthma can be a remitting and fluctuating disease. The diagnosis is not difficult in the classical case, but asthma can remain unrecognised for some time with atypical symptoms.

Characteristic symptoms are an expiratory wheeze, chest tightness and a cough which may be non-productive or produce small amounts of clear, thick, sticky sputum, and dyspnoea. Tenacious plugs of mucus may be expectorated. These symptoms may occur spontaneously and are often worse at night, or they may occur with chest infections, after exercise, with laughter or following foods containing sulphites such as dried fruit, white wine and orange juice. *Variant asthma* is the term sometimes given to asthma with atypical features, particularly coughing and dyspnoea in the absence of wheezing.

Examination in the intervals between symptoms may reveal no abnormalities, or there may be wheezing and prolonged expiration on auscultation. Auscultation is an unreliable indicator of the degree of bronchospasm, and spirometry or peak flow readings are always required as part of the assessment. In acute severe asthma there may be no wheeze, and the most alarming finding is a silent chest where there is little movement of air because of severe bronchoconstriction. With chronic severe and persistent asthma there may be signs of hyperinflation of the chest, with the ribs horizontal and increased antero-posterior diameter. These advanced signs normally should not be encountered in modern practice.

The patient may also have other allergic diseases such as eczema or allergic rhinitis. It is important to document these findings. Firstly, it can characterise the asthma as atopic. Allergic diseases are multisystem and asthma is often only one manifestation, albeit the most important in many cases. Secondly, management requires attention to all aspects of the disease for optimal control of symptoms.

Diagnosis

History is important in eliciting classical symptoms, in determining severity and stability of asthma, the presence of other atopic diseases, and possible precipitants. Physical examination may reveal no abnormal signs in the chest in the interval between episodes of asthma. Even in acute asthma the chest may be ominously quiet, and under these circumstances a silent chest with lack of wheezing is an indication of severity. Investigations are necessary to establish the degree of physiological involvement and to determine the pathogenesis with a view to identifying reversible factors.

Investigations required for diagnosis and elective management

Physiological measurements

There are two simple methods, peak expiratory flow rate (PEFR) using a peak flow meter, or spirometry which indicates forced vital capacity (FVC) and forced expiratory volume in one second (FEV1). Reversibility of airways obstruction is demonstrated by repeating the test 15 minutes after inhalation of a β-2 agonist such as salbutamol or terbutaline. An increase in FEV1 greater than 15% if the baseline FEV1 is greater than 1.3 L, or 20% in PEFR if the baseline is greater than 300 L/min, or if the PEFR varies more than 20% a day on more than one day, is diagnostic of asthma (National Asthma Campaign, 1996). These measurements should form part of every assessment of patients with asthma, just as measurement of blood pressure is necessary in managing patients with hypertension. The findings on examination and physiological measurements may be normal at any one point in time. To overcome this problem the patient can be loaned a peak flow meter to record PEFR in the morning and evening at home over a 1 to 2 week period. Asthmatics characteristically show some variability in daily PEFR, with lower readings being present in the mornings. However, diurnal variation of greater than 25% indicates that asthma is unstable and that the patient is at high risk of life-threatening disease.

It may sometimes be necessary to confirm the diagnosis of asthma by demonstrating the presence of bronchial hyperresponsiveness. This is done by determining the dose of inhaled histamine required to reduce the FEV1 by 20%. This is known as the PD20 of histamine. Figure 12.1 shows typical histamine responses in asthmatics and in patients with varying grades of asthma. This test is a specialist procedure. Other provocative agents can be used such as inhalation of methacholine or hypertonic saline, or exercise.

Investigation of allergic factors

Every asthmatic should undergo assessment to identify potential allergic factors. Therefore, skin prick testing or RASTs should be performed at some stage of their illness, preferably as soon as possible after presentation. It is rarely necessary to perform bronchial provocation studies to establish the role of potential allergens. This measure is most frequently used in the investigation of occupational allergies. It is a specialist procedure and should only be done in a hospital or similar setting.

Other investigations

Radiology may show the presence of associated disease such as consolidation, collapse, fluffy infiltrates of allergic bronchopulmonary aspergillosis, or a fungal ball. The chest x-ray is normal in uncomplicated asthma. However, it should be done when there are unusual clinical features which raise the possibility of some other disease.

Full blood count may show the presence of *eosinophilia*. This does not distinguish between allergic and non-allergic asthma, but eosinophilia reflects the severity of disease. It is hardly ever higher than 1,000 to 2,000/mm^3, even in the most severe asthma, and if higher levels are present another diagnosis should be considered. Assays of eosinophil products in serum, sputum or broncho-alveolar washings are more sensitive indices of severity than is the degree of eosinophilia. Levels of eosinophil cationic protein (ECP) correlate well with other indices of severity such as reduction in FEV1. The

FIGURE 12.1 **Histamine provocation test.** Response to inhalation of increasing doses of histamine.

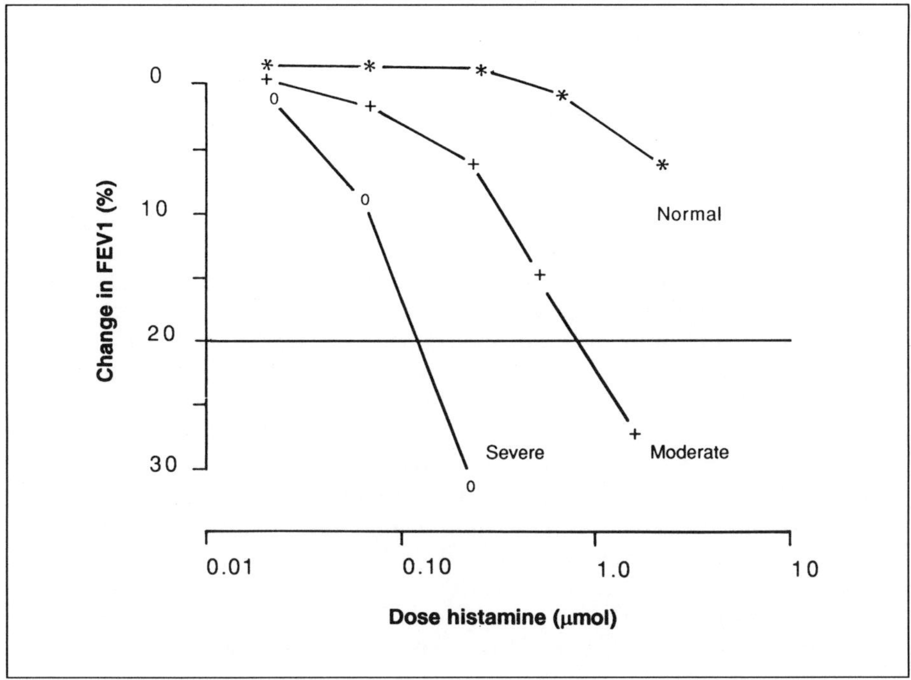

place of these investigations in the clinical management of asthma remains to be determined.

Serum IgE levels are often raised in allergic asthma but are of limited diagnostic significance. However, the finding of very high levels of IgE in asthma should alert one to the possibility of allergic bronchopulmonary aspergillosis. Aspergillus precipitins are present in the serum with aspergillosis and are a useful confirmatory test.

Investigations in acute severe asthma

The preoccupation in management of acute asthma is to achieve improvement in respiratory function and gas exchange, and investigations are directed to establish the degree of severity. *Arterial blood gases* in adults or oximetry in children need to be determined. Hypoxia indicates severity. In moderate cases there is reduced pCO2 because of hyperventilation, and the development of hypercapnia is of serious prognostic significance.

Chest x-ray should always be done if asthma is of sufficient severity to require emergency hospital management, and especially if breath sounds are soft. Pneumothorax can easily be missed under these circumstances and can seriously compromise lung function. Plugging of airways by inspissated mucus can lead to collapse.

Differential diagnosis

Two aphorisms are worth remembering:

1. All that wheezes is not asthma.
2. Asthma does not always wheeze.

Asthma should be distinguished from:

Stridor caused by obstruction to airways. The noise is predominantly inspiratory, whereas in asthma the obstruction is expiratory. In children causes of stridor include croup, bronchiolitis, viral infections and inhalation of a foreign body. In adults stridor may be caused by vocal cord dysfunction, intrabronchial tumours or constriction of major airways by tumour, lymph nodes or mediastinal masses including retrosternal goitre.

Cardiac failure may present with wheezing, hence the historic term 'cardiac asthma'. Left ventricular failure may result in paroxysmal nocturnal dyspnoea which can be mistaken for asthma. The sputum is frothy and often pink.

Pulmonary embolism may be associated with wheezing.

Chronic airways limitation (chronic bronchitis and emphysema). The dyspnoea is clearly of respiratory origin but it is fixed and not reversible with bronchodilators. Sometimes it is difficult to distinguish between these possibilities and they may coexist with an element of reversibility in patients with obstructive airways disease.

Hyperventilation can give rise to dyspnoea and noisy breathing which can be mistaken for asthma. Spirometry during symptomatic periods will indicate that there is no obstruction and no response to bronchodilators.

Acidosis with deep sighing respiration can be mistaken for asthma on occasions.

Recurrent aspiration. This usually implies the presence of some disturbance in swallowing as in cerebrovascular disease.

Cystic fibrosis. Patients may have a wheezy cough but there is usually copious mucopurulent sputum.

Other rare causes of wheezing include pulmonary infiltration with eosinophils (PIE) and pulmonary vasculitis, in particular the Churg Strauss syndrome. These conditions should be suspected if there is an abnormal chest x-ray and a peripheral blood eosinophil count in the thousands. Eosinophilia in asthma is rarely greater than 1,000 to 2,000/mm^3.

Management

The aims of therapy are to:

1. Abolish symptoms and restore normal lung function.
2. Prevent the development of acute attacks of asthma (an acute attack of asthma is an indication of failure of management).
3. Identify and remove potential precipitants.
4. Reverse the pathology of acute asthma, thereby preventing the development of future attacks of asthma and long-term deterioration in lung function.

Interval management

Despite the efficacy of modern drugs, the prevalence of asthma is increasing in many countries in the world. Asthma management plans have been devised in many countries in an attempt to address this problem. The Australian Asthma Management Plan of the National Asthma Campaign (see Further Reading list) has been widely adopted here and there are indications that it has had a positive impact on asthma management.

Asthma is a chronic disease which requires an ongoing relationship between patient and doctor. There should be regular follow-up of all patients with more than mild intermittent symptoms, and the patient should be provided with an asthma management plan.

General management principles

1. *Improve general health.* Such measures have a positive impact on disease management. Attention is paid to:
   (a) good diet and sufficient sleep;
   (b) quality of life issues, including family support and leisure pursuits;
   (c) management of psychological stresses;
   (d) avoidance of cigarettes;
   (e) specific advice about choice of occupations, and/or avoidance of pollutants;
   (f) advice regarding choice of house if the opportunity arises.
2. *Improve functional capacity.* Exercise can induce bronchospasm. However, it is important for asthmatics to maintain a good level of fitness as this improves the efficiency with which they can achieve their physical tasks. Swimming is less likely to induce asthma than running. It is important to do warm-up exercises before vigorous activity. Asthma does not interfere with sporting activity.
3. *Identify and remove precipitating factors.* These include inhaled allergens, as well as other factors such as food intolerance or dealing with exercise-induced asthma. Where there is clear evidence for GERD, this should be treated with appropriate measures which include the use of an H2 antagonist or omeprazole, and in infants, measures such as thickened feeds and a more upright position after feeding.
4. *Treatment of associated allergic symptoms.* Rhinitis can have a significant

TABLE 12.5 **The six steps of the asthma management plan**

1. Assess asthma severity when not in acute attack.
2. Achieve best lung function.
3. Avoid trigger factors to maintain best lung function.
4. Optimal medication to maintain best lung function.
5. Develop a written action plan.
6. Educate and review regularly.

(Adapted from *Asthma Management Handbook 1996*. National Asthma Campaign, Melbourne).

impact on good asthma control, and nasal corticosteroids and anti-histamines may be required. Contrary to earlier teaching it is now accepted that there is no contra-indication to the use of antihistamines in asthma.

5. *Follow-up.* This is important to identify deterioration in asthma control as early as possible. This is suggested by waking at night with asthma, increasing symptoms such as cough and dyspnoea, increased usage of bronchodilators, failure of brochodilators to relieve symptoms, increased diurnal variation in peak flow readings and falling peak flow. With a written asthma plan the patient knows in advance the correct course of action which can be followed without delay.

6. *Exercise-induced asthma.* This may indicate undertreatment and the need for increasing medication. It can be prevented by premedication with inhaled β-2 agonists, sodium cromoglycate or nedocromil sodium.

7. *Immunotherapy.* There may be a role in carefully selected patients. Its prescription must be regarded as a specialist procedure and this is particularly the case in asthma (see Chapter 7).

Principles of drug use in asthma

Management principles have changed significantly in the past decade. Whereas previously the objective of management was to achieve bronchodilation, modern treatment aims to reverse the allergic inflammation which is the basis of the asthmatic reaction. This means that inhaled anti-inflammatory agents are used early in management.

In mild episodic asthma where episodes occur less frequently than once a week and are easily reversed with inhaled bronchodilators, it is sufficient to use short-acting inhaled bronchodilators as required. However, in all but the mildest cases, and if bronchodilators are necessary more frequently, preventive therapy with sodium cromoglycate, inhaled corticosteroids or nedocromil sodium should be started with inhaled bronchodilators being used for symptoms.

Persistent severe asthma requires regular anti-inflammatory treatment with high-dose inhaled corticosteroids, with or without inhaled sodium cromoglycate or nedocromil sodium. Bronchodilators are used as required. If there is troublesome nocturnal asthma, addition of long-acting bronchodilators such as salmeterol can be considered. Systemic corticosteroids may be required for uncontrolled symptoms or deterioration.

Acute severe asthma

Initial assessment is performed as rapidly as possible in order to obtain essential information and so as not to delay initiation of effective therapy. A decision needs to be taken early as to whether the patient needs to be admitted to hospital. This is determined by the severity of the disease.

Pharmacological agents

More details are given in Chapters 4 and 6.

Beta-2 agonists cause bronchodilation with immediate relief of symptoms

TABLE 12.6 **Criteria for severity of acute asthma**

	Mild	**Moderate**	**Severe**
Talks in	Sentences	Phrases	Words
Exhausted	No	No	Yes
Altered consciousness	No	No	Yes
Pulse rate	<100/min	100–120/min	>120/min
Pulsus paradoxus	No	No	Yes, especially children
Intensity of wheeze	Audible	Loud	Soft
Breath sounds	Prolonged expiration or normal	Wheeze	May be soft
PEFR (% predicted)	>60%	40–60%	<40% or <100 L/min
FEV_1 (% predicted)	>60%	40–60%	<40% or <1 L
Arterial pO2	Not necessary	>60 mmHg	<60 mmHg
Arterial pCO2	Not necessary	<40 mmHg	>40 mmHg

TABLE 12.7 **Which patients should go to hospital?**

- Acute asthma of moderate or severe grade (see Table 12.6)
- No improvement despite adequate bronchodilation
- As dictated by written personal asthma management plan
- A known unfavourable pattern of attack
- Rapid, sudden, unexpected deterioration

and in all but the mildest, intermittent cases, regular inhaled corticosteroids are the primary agents. Excessive and increasing usage of β-2 agonists indicates that therapy is inadequate and there is a need for more intensive anti-inflammatory treatment. Agents presently in common usage are salbutamol and terbutaline. Long-acting agents such as salmeterol are becoming available and are indicated for prolonged bronchodilation, for example to prevent nocturnal asthma. They are not anti-inflammatory and do not substitute for agents such as inhaled corticosteroids which must be continued in adequate doses. They should not be used for acute relief of symptoms or in the management of acute severe asthma.

Anti-inflammatory agents are indicated in all but the mildest and most intermittent cases of asthma. *Inhaled corticosteroids* are now considered first-line treatment in adults with moderate to severe, frequent or persistent asthma. In the majority of patients adequate doses can be provided by inhalation without the side effects which accompany oral or parenteral administration. Available preparations include:

Beclomethasone diproprionate, available in 50, 100 and 250 mcg doses per activation. Agents can be administered by metered dose aerosols, with the use of a spacer device, or in solution to be used in a nebuliser.

TABLE 12.8 **Management of acute asthma**

	Mild	Moderate	Severe
Admission to hospital	No	Probable	Yes—acute/intensive care
Oxygen	At least 8 L/min for inspired oxygen concentration of 50%. Monitor by oximetry		
Nebulised β-agonist	1 ml 0.5% salbutamol +3 ml saline	2 ml 0.5% salbutamol +2 ml saline 1–4 hourly	2 ml 0.5% salbutamol +2 ml saline every 15–30 mins. Give salbutamol IV if no response
Nebulised ipratropium	No	Optional	2 ml 0.025% 2 hourly
Corticosteroids			
Oral prednisone	Possible	Yes. Starting 60–80 mg daily	No
IV hydrocortisone	No	200 mg stat	200 mg 6 hourly for 24 hours then review
Aminophylline	Of uncertain benefit with maximal β-2 agonists		IV an alternative to IV salbutamol
Adrenaline	No	No	0.5 ml subcutaneously or IMI if part of anaphylaxis
Observations	Regular	Continuous	Continuous

(Adapted from *Asthma Management Handbook 1996*. National Asthma Campaign, Melbourne).

Budesonide, available as a metered dose aerosol or through a Turbuhaler. The latter is a particularly efficient delivery system. Doses are 50, 100, 200 and 400 mcg per dose.

Fluticasone diproprionate. This is a more potent inhaled corticosteroid which is intended for those patients on high-dose inhaled corticosteroids who are experiencing corticosteroid side effects. It is administered through a metered dose aerosol or with a self-activating disc delivery system. Doses are 50, 100 and 250 mcg per dose. Any drug absorbed through the gastrointestinal system undergoes extensive first pass hepatic metabolism so that there is little opportunity for systemic effects. At the present time it is indicated for treatment of patients on maximal doses of inhaled corticosteroids who are experiencing systemic effects. Equivalent efficacy is achieved at lower doses and with less systemic absorption.

Oral or parenteral administration of steroids are required for exacerbations of asthma, despite maximal doses of inhaled corticosteroids. Steroid resistance can arise as a result of the concomitant use of beta-blocking agents, because of continuing exposure to allergen, or in rare instances of intrinsic steroid resistance, the mechanism of which is poorly understood.

Sodium cromoglycate is particularly useful in childhood asthma. It is also an effective agent for preventing exercise-induced bronchospasm if used 15 minutes before the start of exercise.

Nedocromil sodium is an effective alternative in mild to moderate asthma as an anti-inflammatory agent on its own, or as a steroid sparing agent. The usual dose is two puffs (4 mg) two to four times daily.

Other anti-inflammatory agents include *immunosuppressives* such as cyclosporine, methotrexate and oral gold. The rationale for their use is that they reduce the infiltration of Th2 cells which are involved in the pathogenesis of asthma. Their use should be regarded as experimental and confined to specialists.

Theophylline used to be widely used as adjunct to beta-adrenergic agonists, but its use is now largely limited to patients who are poorly controlled on multiple medications or who have been on these agents for long periods of time. Sustained release preparations are preferable. Their therapeutic index is low, i.e. there is little discrimination between therapeutic and toxic levels. Levels are influenced by several drug interactions, for example erythromycin and cimetidine. Serum levels should be performed while establishing the appropriate dosage. Intravenous aminophylline for treatment of acute severe asthma is used infrequently and is mainly of historic interest.

Anticholinergic agents. Ipratropium bromide is an atropine-like drug which has an additive effect to beta-adrenergic agents. It is particularly useful in asthma when chronic bronchitis with sputum production is also present.

Adrenaline is the drug of choice for management of anaphylaxis. It is indicated where asthma is part of the syndrome of anaphylaxis, where anaphylaxis has occurred previously, and for precipitous asthma attacks such as may occur after adverse reactions to food ingestion. Self-administration preparations are available including Min-I-Jet and Epi-Pen.

Prognosis—natural history of asthma

Childhood asthma

Parents are often told that many children with asthma will go into remission at puberty. The evidence on this point is unclear. It appears that about 50% of children with mild intermittent asthma will 'grow out of it' by adulthood, but it will persist in those with more severe disease. Socio-economic factors play a role in the prognosis. In the USA black children and those from inner city homes are less likely to go into remission.

In adults

The natural history of asthma is poorly documented in adults. Recent studies suggest that removal from exposure to allergens will, over a long period of time, lead to a reduction in bronchial hyperresponsiveness. It is also possible that in the future modern approaches to immunotherapy may be more effective and again could lead to reduced bronchial hyperresponsiveness.

When to refer to a specialist

1. All asthmatics deserve full investigation of possible allergic factors at an early stage of their illness. This requires a detailed history supplemented by investigations for allergic factors, using skin prick tests in particular. If this is not feasible in a general practice setting, the patient should be referred to an appropriate specialist or hospital clinic with expertise in identifying and treating allergic conditions and asthma.

TABLE 12.9 **Patients at risk of dying from asthma**

Clinical features
1. Hospital admission for asthma in the past 12 months.
2. Frequent need for emergency treatment of asthma in the past 12 months.
3. Previous admission to intensive care or near-fatal attack of asthma.
4. Excessive use of inhaled bronchodilators. Canister lasts less than 3 weeks.
5. Associated food allergy (often with sudden acute episodes of asthma).
6. Aspirin or NSAID hypersensitivity.
7. Denial of asthma, especially teenagers.
8. Poor compliance with therapy, failure to follow-up.
9. Lack of perception of symptoms when physiological measurements are poor.
10. Nocturnal asthma.
11. Marked diurnal variation (>25% variation in PEFR).

Psychosocial factors
1. Economically disadvantaged.
2. Inadequate medical attention.
3. Personal psychological problems, e.g. depression.

2. The patient should be referred to a specialist where there are indications of poor control or unstable asthma, i.e. increasing bronchodilator usage (more than four usages in a 24 hour period), wakening at night from asthma, or persisting symptoms of wheeze, cough or dyspnoea despite optimal therapy.

3. The patient should be referred to a specialist when there are episodes of sudden deterioration in lung function or sudden onset of symptoms. The possibility of reactions to foods must be considered.

Background

Asthma is an inflammatory disease of the airways characterised by the appearance of large numbers of eosinophils, to the extent that the term 'eosinophilic bronchitis' has been given to the disease (Barnes PJ. Asthma as an axon reflex. *Lancet* 1986; 1: 242). This inflammation is responsible for the characteristic hyperresponsiveness of bronchi in asthma to a variety of non-specific stimuli. Until recently many people believed that asthma was predominantly a disorder of the pulmonary airways and that allergy had no role to play. This arose from observations that allergic factors were triggers for acute asthma in only up to 50% of cases, and that other factors such as viral infections in children were more important triggers. It was also difficult to understand how the immediate IgE mediated response could explain the chronic inflammatory nature of asthma. However, with an understanding of the role of the late allergic response came an appreciation of the possible role of allergy in asthma.

Pathology of asthma

Bronchial biopsies from asthmatics have been studied in various stages of their disease. Tissue from airways of mild asthmatics have been obtained during the course of investigations for other pathology, or at necropsy following accidental death. Tissue from airways of patients dying in status asthmaticus are also available for study.

In severe disease the lumen is occluded with inspissated mucus which can form casts of the bronchial tubes and when coughed up may be spiral or have the shape of the airway—the so-called Curshmann spirals. The mucus contains numerous eosinophils and the crystalline cytoplasmic components of eosinophils known as Charcot Leyden crystals. Eosinophil products such as eosinophil cationic protein (ECP) can be measured in bronchial lavage and in peripheral blood and give a measure of severity of the disease.

Airway narrowing results from oedema of the bronchial wall and surrounding tissues, and from hypertrophy of bronchial wall smooth musculature. The mucosal lining is damaged with stripping of cells and exposure of nerve endings. Goblet cells are increased in number. The basement membrane is thickened and there is fibrosis in the more chronic cases.

Inflammatory changes in the submucosa are characterised by the presence of oedema and prominent eosinophils, as well as lymphocytes, macrophages, fibroblasts and neutrophils. Lymphocytes are CD4+ T helper

FIGURE 12.2 **Pathology of the asthmatic airway.**
Photomicrograph of a bronchus from a patient dying in status asthmaticus. (**a**) Low power, showing occlusion of the lumen with mucus plug, stripping of epithelial lining, hypertrophy of bronchial muscle, congestion, oedema and infiltration of inflammatory cells (haematoxylin and eosin ×20). (**b**) High power detail of inflammatory infiltrate with prominence of eosinophils and thickening of basement membrane (haematoxylin and eosin ×400).

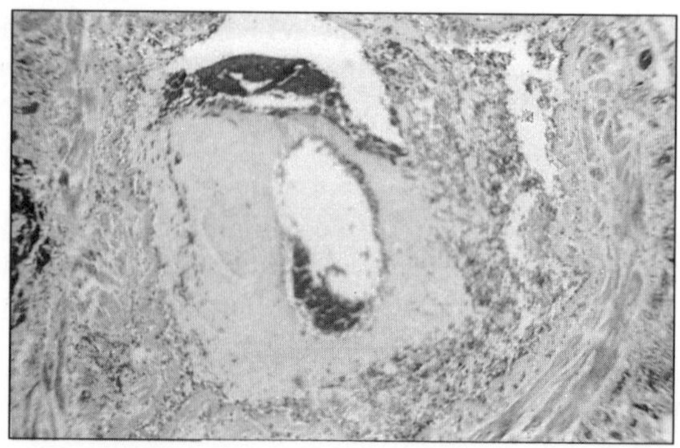

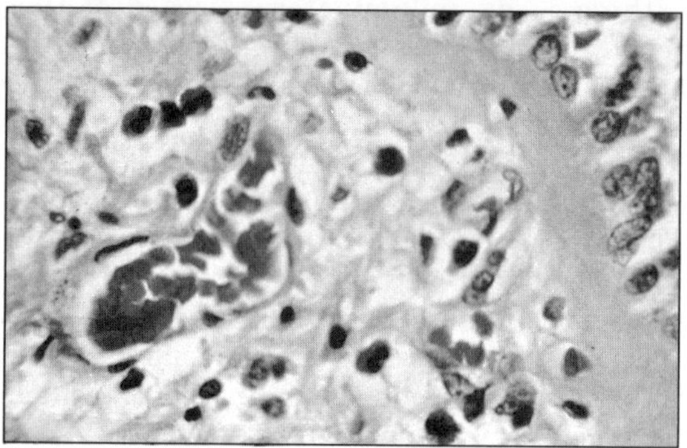

cells of the Th2 type. The elastic lamina may be disrupted in places, and in long-standing cases there are secondary changes of fibrosis. In intervals between attacks and with inhaled corticosteroid the changes resolve but thickening of basement membrane persists.

Pathogenesis

Immunology

Contact with the relevant allergen in the sensitised individual results in release of preformed mediators, including histamine and bradykinin, and the formation and release of arachidonic acid metabolites, especially the leukotrienes (LT) C4, D4 and E4 previously known as slow reacting substance of anaphylaxis (SRS-A), and platelet activating factor (PAF). These powerful bronchoconstrictors cause contraction of bronchial smooth muscle resulting in a drop in FEV1 in 15 to 20 minutes, the immediate response. This is reversed with β-2 agonists. This corresponds with the acute bronchoconstriction following allergen challenge in the natural situation and with provocation. However, it does not account for the persistent symptoms and chronic nature of asthma, nor for the inflammation which is characteristic of this disease.

Some 4 to 6 hours after exposure to allergen there is a second, more

FIGURE 12.3 **The bronchoconstrictor response to inhaled allergen
challenge in an allergic individual.**

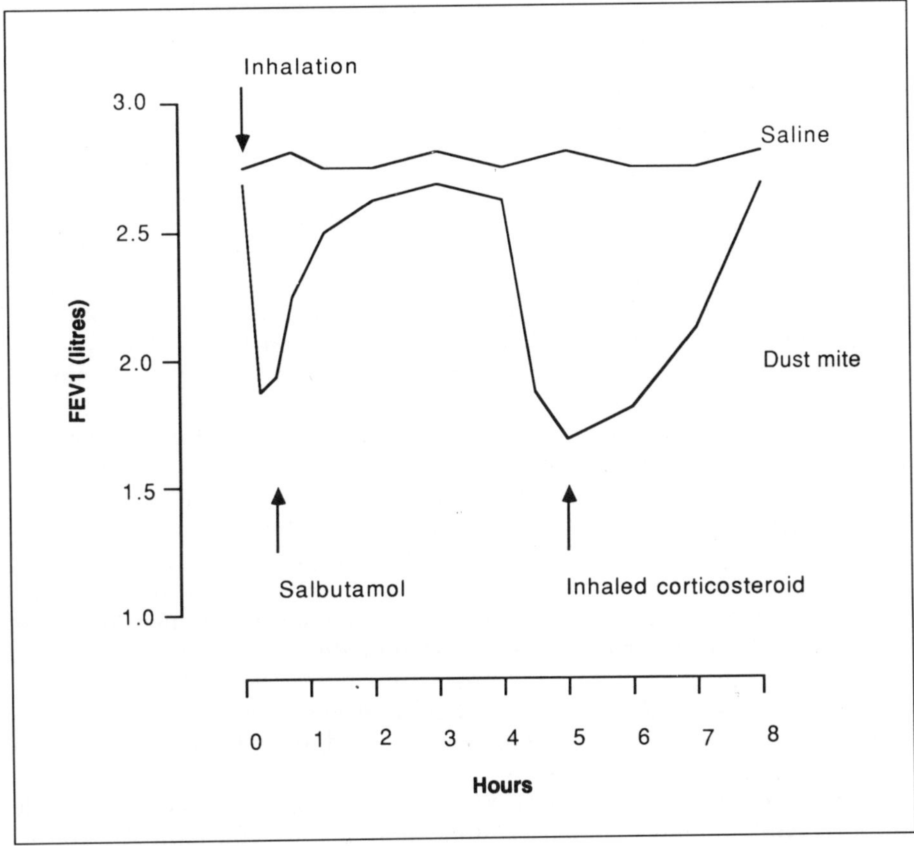

sustained reduction in FEV1 known as the late allergic reaction (LAR). This
is accompanied by the typical allergic inflammatory reaction in bronchi. The
inflammatory response is brought about by recruitment and activation of Th2
cells and release of newly formed mediators from mast cells. Expansion of the
Th2 population is favoured by release of the cytokine IL-4 from mast cells and
Th2 cells, and by nitric oxide (NO) production which down-regulates Th1
with reduced interferon gamma IFN-γ production and secondary up-regula-
tion of Th2 cells. Mast cells release mediators which include the leukotrienes
LTC4, LTD4 and LTE4 which were previously known as slow-reacting substance of anaphylaxis and which are responsible for smooth muscle contraction and increased vascular permeability; LTB4 which is chemotactic for
inflammatory cells; and prostaglandin PGD2 which causes vasodilatation
and smooth muscle contraction. Other cytokines increase cell adhesion molecule expression which allow leucocytes to leave the circulation and enter
inflammatory sites in tissues. Biopsies of asthmatic bronchi show increased
numbers of CD4+ Th2 cells in the submucosa and there is some evidence that

the severity of the asthma coincides with the numbers of these cells in the bronchial wall. Eosinophils release highly toxic biological products which strip off the epithelium and expose underlying nerve endings which are stimulated by histamine.

Role of the nervous system

The dramatic and widespread response to a few molecules of allergen can only reasonably be explained on the basis of neurological amplification of the stimulus. The best illustration of this reaction is the development of anaphylaxis following allergen exposure, and intense bronchospasm can be an integral part of the syndrome. There is evidence that lodgement of allergen in upper airways can provoke an asthmatic reaction through a nasobronchial reflex, although the evidence for this is not universally accepted. However, it would explain why allergenic particles which are too large to enter terminal respiratory bronchioles can induce an asthmatic reaction.

There are many clues to the involvement of neurological mechanisms in asthma. The effects of psychological factors on precipitating asthma have been appreciated for a long time. It is being increasingly realised that there is an intimate interaction between immunological and nervous systems which operate in both directions. Lymphocytes bear receptors for neurotransmitters and some central nervous system cells have surface proteins similar to those of lymphocytes. It is known that neurovascular reflexes play an important role in inflammatory changes in the skin, and immunological stimulation leads to increased excitability of nerves innervating airways. Before modern effective drugs became available it was found that section of appropriate nerves could lead to improvement in intractible asthma.

The nervous system has been known for a long time to be responsible for maintaining bronchial muscle tone and airway function. The *parasympathetic* system is 'excitatory' through the vagus nerve to small airways. The major neurotransmitter is acetylcholine which is responsible for causing bronchoconstriction and mucus secretion. There is little, if any, *sympathetic* innervation of the airways in man. However, there are large numbers of both α-adrenergic and β-adrenergic receptors in the lung, with β-2 predominating. The sympathetic system is 'inhibitory' in that β-2 receptors mediate smooth muscle relaxation, inhibit mast cell mediator release and decrease cholinergic neurotransmission. The role of α-adrenergic receptors is less clear. Alpha-1 receptors have weak broncho-constrictor effects, increase mucus secretion and increase mast cell mediator release. Alpha-2 receptors inhibit cholinergic and non-cholinergic transmission.

A third system, the *non-adrenergic-non-cholinergic* (NANC) pathway is important in controlling airway function. Because of the lack of direct sympathetic innervation, the non-adrenergic pathway is probably the most important inhibitory bronchodilator influence. Its effects are mediated by the neuropeptides, VIP (vasoactive intestinal peptide) and PHM (peptide histidine methionine). The excitatory transmitters of the non-cholinergic pathway are the tachykinins, which include substance P, neurokinin A and

B, and calcitonin gene related peptide (CGRP). Capsaicin is an agonist for tachykinin receptors and can destroy them. Stimulation of these capsaicin sensitive receptors leads to bronchospasm with increased protein extravasation and this is an important up-regulator of inflammatory responses. Nitric oxide is an important transmitter or modulator in the NANC system.

It has been suggested for many years that asthmatics have altered autonomic function which contributes to a tendency to bronchoconstriction and increased mucus secretion resulting in bronchial hyperresponsiveness. More than 30 years ago Szentivanyi described partial blockade of the β-adrenergic receptor in atopy so that it was less receptive to β-agonists. Beta-blocking agents convert partial into complete blockade and are contraindicated in asthma and in patients who are undergoing desensitisation. These drugs cause severe bronchospasm and aggravate allergic reactions and anaphylaxis which become difficult if not impossible to reverse.

Role of infections in asthma

Viral infections are the most common precipitants of acute asthma in infants and children. Respiratory syncytial virus (RSV) is most commonly involved, but parainfluenza, influenza and rhinoviruses have also been implicated. In older children mycoplasma infection is a similar problem, but bacterial infections do not seem to have the same effect. Viral infections are less troublesome in adults. There are several explanations for the association between viral infection and the development of bronchospasm and asthma. Viral infections are more likely to precipitate wheezing in atopic subjects. Virus specific IgE levels are higher in these children after an infection, and there is circumstantial evidence that it contributes to mediator release and the pathogenesis of asthma. Furthermore, the presence of high RSV-IgE antibody titres predicts the likelihood of future wheezing episodes after an initial episode of bronchiolitis. Viral infection can also affect airway function and damage bronchial epithelium, leading to bronchial hyperresponsiveness. It can affect the immune system in several ways. Gamma-interferon production is increased, resulting in activation of eosinophils and basophils and expression of adhesion molecules. The major human receptor for rhinovirus is ICAM-1, an adhesion molecule on the surface of endothelial cells, fibroblasts, lymphocytes and monocytes. Its natural ligand is LFA-1 which is found on leucocytes, including T-cells. By binding to these molecules viral infections can interfere with cell function and traffic, increasing the inflammatory process and epithelial damage. Viral infections also alter β-adrenergic function and enhance cholinergic sensitivity, thereby increasing bronchial hyperresponsiveness.

Further reading

Asthma Management Handbook 1996. National Asthma Campaign Ltd, Melbourne.

Bochner BS, Undem BJ, Lichtenstein LM. Immunological aspects of allergic asthma. *In:* Paul WE, Fathman CG, Metzger H (eds). *Annu Rev Immunol*. Palo Alto: Annual Reviews Inc, 1994; 12: 295–335.

Rees J, Price J. ABC of asthma. 3rd ed. Nedlands WA: BMJ Publishing Group, AMAS Medical Publications, 1995.

Chapter 13

Other immunological diseases of the lung

Allergic bronchopulmonary aspergillosis (ABPA)

Introduction

Aspergillus is a ubiquitous saprophyte, normally colonising airways and not producing any disease. However, it can produce disease in several ways. It can give rise to allergic asthma due to IgE mediated reactions. In chronic, severe, usually steroid-dependent asthma, hyphae persist in bronchial airways and give rise to allergic bronchopulmonary aspergillosis (ABPA). If large numbers of spores are inhaled it can induce extrinsic allergic alveolitis. In immuno-incompetent patients it can become invasive, produce pneumonia, abscesses and disseminated disease. It can colonise abscess and bronchiectatic cavities and produce aspergillomas, usually in a non-atopic patient.

Clinical presentation of ABPA

The usual patient has severe chronic steroid-dependent asthma or is receiving large doses of inhaled corticosteroids. The condition is suspected when there is worsening asthma, and with the appearance on chest x-ray of fluffy infiltrative changes which were not present previously. The patient may develop a productive cough and expectorate brownish plugs, and may have flu-like symptoms and a fever. This is one condition where measurement of serum IgE levels is of great value. Serum IgE is very high, usually over 1,000 Ku/L. An increase over a previous reading is of diagnostic value, and levels tend to fall with treatment which can be helpful in monitoring progress of the disease. The patient may have an eosinophilia. Sputum examination may reveal eosinophils and aspergillus hyphae. Untreated, there is progressive tissue damage leading to proximal bronchiectasis.

Management

High doses of oral steroids are required, in the order of 40 to 60 mg prednisone per day over several weeks, reducing to a lower maintenance dose for a 3 month period. Inhaled corticosteroids are ineffective.

Hypersensitivity pneumonitis

Immune complex deposition and cell mediated immune reactions to extrinsic antigens can give rise to a number of diseases of the lung.

Extrinsic allergic alveolitis

The classical clinical features are of a cough, often non-productive, with dyspnoea, myalgia and temperature. A careful history may reveal the onset of symptoms about 4 to 6 hours after exposure to antigen. However, this pattern of symptoms may not be obvious where the patient has continuous or repeated contact with the antigen. Instead, symptoms may be progressive with chronic cough, dyspnoea and reduced exercise tolerance. Physical examination reveals widespread fine crepitations. Chest x-ray shows a diffuse parenchymal pattern with reticular and nodular shadowing. Blood gases show reduced pO_2 and pCO_2, indicating a diffusion defect and compensatory hyperventilation. Chronic exposure will lead to secondary irreversible changes with pulmonary fibrosis. Investigations reveal the presence of IgG precipitating antibody to the relevant antigen. The antibody may be present in the absence of disease, so in itself it does not make the diagnosis, although it is necessary for the diagnosis.

Management

It is most important to identify the offending antigen and to remove it from the environment. Table 13.1 shows the common antigens involved in this disease. Oral steroids are required to suppress the inflammatory reaction. Once fibrosis has occurred the changes are irreversible.

TABLE 13.1 **Common antigens involved in extrinsic allergic alveolitis**

Antigen	Source of antigen	Disease
Avian proteins	Bird droppings, feathers	Pigeon breeder's lung
	Pigeons, budgerigars, canaries	Bird fancier's lung
Micro-organisms including fungi		
Thermophilic	Mouldy hay and grain	Farmer's lung
actinomycetes including	Mushroom compost	Mushroom picker's lung
Micropolyspora species	Contaminated water systems	Humidifier pneumonitis
Aspergillus clavatus	Mouldy barley	Malt worker's lung
Penicillium casei	Cheese mould	Cheese washer's lung
Industrial chemicals		
Phthalic anhydride	Epoxy resin	Epoxy resin worker's lung
Toluene diisocyanate	Paint catalyst	Porcelain worker's lung
Trimellitic anhydride	Plastics industry	Plastic worker's lung

Further reading

Fink JN. Hypersensitivity pneumonitis. *In:* Middleton Jnr E, Reed CE, Ellis EF, Adkinson NF, Yunginger JW, Busse WW (eds). Allergy. Principles and Practice. 4th Ed. St Louis, USA: Mosby, 1993; 1415–31.

Slavin RG. Allergic bronchopulmonary aspergillosis. *Clin Rev Allergy* 1985; 3: 167.

Chapter 14

Atopic eczema

Introduction

Atopic eczema, also known as atopic dermatitis, is one of the most common and troublesome skin conditions presenting to the doctor. In common with other allergic conditions its prevalence has increased over the past 25 years from 3 to 4% of the childhood population in the 1960s to around 13% in the 1980s. The prevalence declines rapidly with approach of adulthood. It was first described by Besnier and Brocq in 1885 and became known as Besnier's prurigo in Europe, a name which is still used in European literature. It is known also by a number of other names which are descriptive of some of its characteristics, such as neurodermatitis, infantile eczema and flexoral eczema.

Definition

Eczema and dermatitis are interchangeable terms, although the term dermatitis is sometimes used to embrace all forms of skin inflammation, while eczema is taken to mean a particular form of dermatitis.

Classification

Eczema has been divided into *endogenous (constitutional)* and *exogenous* forms, but this division is artificial in that extrinsic factors operate in the

TABLE 14.1 **Classification of eczemas**

Endogenous (constitutional) eczema	*Exogenous eczema*
Atopic eczema	Contact dermatitis/eczema
Seborrhoeic dermatitis	allergic
Asteatotic eczema (eczema craquelee) in	irritant
the elderly	Photosensitivity dermatitis/eczema
Pompholyx	Venous eczema
Lichen simplex chronicus	Dermatophyte infection
Eczema associated with systemic disease	

endogenous form, for example atopic eczema, and genetic predisposition probably plays a role in exogenous eczema.

Since age is one important factor determining the distribution and manifestations of the lesions, atopic eczema is also commonly classified as infantile, from about 4 to 6 weeks after birth to 2 years of age, childhood eczema, from 4 to 10 years of age, and adolescent and adult eczema.

Clinical features

Eczema is a particular type of inflammatory condition of the skin characterised clinically by itching, diffuse redness and papules, scaling, and weeping from fissures and vesicles. Atopic eczema has a characteristic distribution depending on the age of the patient. There is frequently thickening of the epidermal layers of the skin known as lichenification, brought about by scratching and rubbing the skin. Eczema is particularly susceptible to secondary bacterial infection and this is often indicated by the presence of scaling, weeping and crusting, and especially by the presence of pustules. Herpes simplex may occasionally be misdiagnosed as bacterial infection. There is also increased susceptibility to fungal infection which can cause the disease to flare. Eczema is a common manifestation of severe atopic disease and often keeps company with other atopic diseases such as asthma and allergic rhinitis.

FIGURE 14.1 **Distribution of eczema in infants and in adults.**

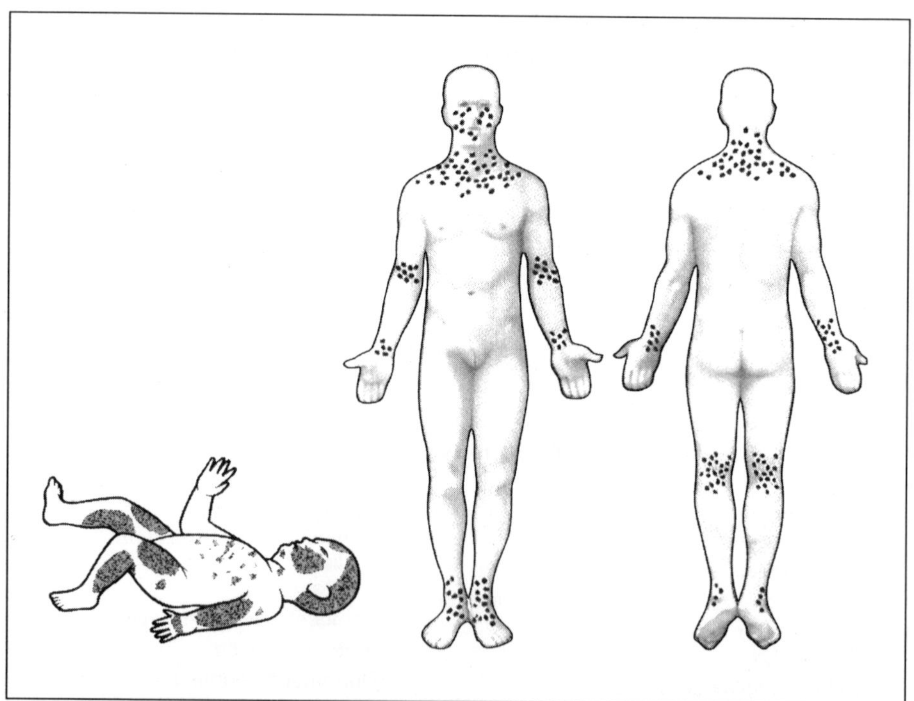

(Reproduced with permission from Allergy and the Skin. Hayfever and Allergy Information Service).

1. *Infantile eczema.* The usual distribution is the face, torso anteriorly, over the back, and extensor surfaces of the limbs and the groin. The nappy area is spared. The skin of the face is red, dry and excoriated, crusted and weeping. The infant is irritable, restless and crying from the itching which often disturbs sleep and may interfere with feeding. There may be scratch marks. Other features are perioral pallor, an extra fold of skin below the lower eyelid, known as Dennie's line, and increased palmar markings. Figure 14.1 shows the classical distribution of the lesions.

2. *Childhood and adult eczema.* These can be considered together since the distribution is similar. The flexures, especially antecubital and popliteal fossae, and the back of the neck are particularly affected. There is often more thickening or lichenification due to rubbing and scratching, than in infants. The lesions are dry but where the skin is broken there is weeping of serous fluid. The skin tends to crack and bleed, especially over knuckles. The distribution on the face tends to involve the circumoral and peri-orbital areas. The uninvolved skin is also often dry (xerosis). There is a tendency to remission as the child approaches adulthood but the more severe forms may persist, sometimes with more localised distribution such as around hands or legs and may be more nummular or resemble lichen simplex chronicus. The palmar skin may be reddened, shiny and thin. There are increased skin markings. In severely affected adults the skin of the face may appear thickened and pale. Eczema can be acute and gener-alised, giving rise to a generalised redness of the skin.

Diagnosis and investigation

Eczema is a clinical diagnosis based on the appearance of the lesions, their distribution and the presence of other atopic features. Criteria for the diagno-sis of atopic eczema have been put forward by the United Kingdom Working Party on Atopic Dermatitis. These are the presence of an itchy skin condition (or parental report of scratching and rubbing in an infant), plus three or more of the following:

1. History of characteristic distribution of the lesions—folds of elbows, be-hind knees, fronts of ankles or around neck (including cheeks of children under the age of 10).
2. Features of atopy—personal history of asthma or hayfever, or if the child is under 4 years of age, atopic disease in a first degree relative.
3. History of general dry skin in the past year.
4. Visible eczema involving flexures, or under the age of 4 years, involving cheeks, forehead and outer limbs.
5. Onset under the age of 2 years if the child is over 4 years of age.

Differential diagnosis

In infants the condition needs to be distinguished from nappy rash, seborrhoeic dermatitis, candidal infection (thrush), and scabies.

In adults and children, consider the following:

Scabies. Itching is intense, and there may be crusting and secondary infection. The distribution of the lesions is characteristic, involving the webs of fingers and toes, flexor aspects of wrists, nipples and groins. The distribution is atypical in infants and may be generalised. The diagnosis can be confirmed by extracting an organism from a burrow with a needle and inspecting it under a microscope. It is always important to enquire whether other members of the family are also involved.

Candidal infection (intertrigo).

Contact dermatitis. Patients with atopic eczema are more prone to develop contact dermatitis and the two conditions may co-exist. Where contact dermatitis is widespread it may be difficult to distinguish from atopic eczema, but the distribution with, for example involvement of flexoral areas, will usually provide the clue.

Lichen simplex chronicus (localised neurodermatitis). There are localised plaques of thickened scaly skin due to persistent rubbing and irritation. It commonly affects ankles, wrists, elbows, knees and occipital areas.

Venous eczema over varicose veins. The distribution is characteristic.

Psoriasis can sometimes cause confusion, although the distribution is usually characteristic, involving extensor surfaces, scalp and peri-umbilical areas.

Photosensitivity. Drugs and locally applied preparations are the most common causes but occasionally an underlying disease such as systemic lupus erythematosus or porphyria may be responsible.

Pompholyx is a relapsing, vesicular lesion affecting the palms, of unknown aetiology but possibly related to psychological factors.

Red man syndrome. Diffuse lymphocyte infiltration by lymphoma can give rise to a picture similar to diffuse severe eczema but it is rare when compared with the frequency of atopic eczema. T cell lymphomas are particularly likely to involve the skin. Sezary's syndrome, due to a malignant proliferation of CD4+ T cells, classically presents with the red man syndrome. The diagnosis is apparent on skin biopsy and sometimes lymphocytes with a characteristic convoluted appearance, the Sezary cells, are present in peripheral blood.

Erisipelas. This is a rapidly spreading, erythematous, red lesion associated with fever and constitutional illness.

TABLE 14.2 **Photosensitising agents**

Drugs administered systemically
  Antimicrobials
    Tetracyclines
    Sulphonamides
    Non-steroidal anti-inflammatory agents, e.g. ibuprofen, piroxicam
  Psoralens
  Phenothiazines, e.g. promethazine

Topical applications
  Fragrances
  Psoralens

In patients with recent onset or deterioration in eczema, especially in association with contact dermatitis of the hands and in high risk groups, always consider the possibility of *latex allergy* (see Chapter 21).

Severe eczema can be associated with a number of immunodeficiency diseases in infancy which, although rare, should be considered especially when there are atypical features.

Precipitating and exacerbating factors

Eczema is a multifactorial disease and in any one patient there may be a number of aggravating factors. These include:

Food allergy. This is more likely in infants and young children than in adults. Foods which are frequently incriminated include milk, eggs, strawberries, fish, peanuts, nuts and soya.

Food additives. Colouring agents and preservatives may exacerbate eczema in susceptible patients.

Inhalant allergens. Occasional patients find that their symptoms deteriorate in spring when pollens are about, or when they are heavily exposed to house dust.

Contact allergens. Deterioration in atopic eczema can result from exposure to contact allergens, for example contact with household pets, allergy to topical medications, or reactions to contact with foods during their preparation. Heavy exposure to house dust mite is considered by many to exacerbate eczema, probably through direct contact with skin, although a role for inhaled or even ingested allergen cannot be ruled out.

Secondary infection. Eczematous skin is highly susceptible to secondary infection, usually by staphylococcus, and this can lead to severe deterioration. It is not always readily recognised. Telltale signs are crusting, vesicles (especially if pustular) and nodules.

Stress. The relationship between flares of eczema and a variety of stresses has been well established.

Irritants. Clothes made of man-made fibres tend not to 'breathe' and may cause considerable discomfort and deterioration in eczema. Some patients find wool is prickly and irritating. Lanolin in wool may also cause sensitisation.

Heat. Hot weather, overheating in bed, hot showers or baths and exercise can lead to deterioration in eczema.

Dry air such as in air-conditioned environments or with heaters in winter.

Investigations

Allergy investigations are required to confirm the diagnosis in difficult cases and to identify allergens which may be responsible for aggravating the condition.

Full blood count frequently shows eosinophilia. In the absence of other causes, a marked neutrophil leucocytosis should alert one to the possibility of secondary bacterial infection of the skin.

Serum IgE levels are raised in over 80% of patients with atopic eczema and levels tend to be higher than in other atopic diseases. The level does not carry any prognostic or therapeutic implications.

Specific IgE antibodies to inhalants and to food allergens can be detected by skin prick testing or RASTs. In severe eczema it may be difficult to find sufficient areas of normal skin to perform these tests or the patient may be taking antihistamines which interfere with them. RASTs are the preferred investigation in these circumstances. Strongly positive RASTs to foods may suggest which challenges should be undertaken and help to define a suitable elimination diet. A strong reaction to house dust mite alerts one to the possibility that it may be contributing to the illness.

Quantitation of immunoglobulins may show selective deficiency of IgA but more commonly IgA levels tend to be raised. The IgG4 subclass of IgG may be raised in atopic eczema, but this is of no practical significance. Patients with long-standing chronic eczema often have a polyclonal increase in gamma globulin due to chronic immune stimulation. These investigations do not help with diagnosis of the condition but may be useful in determining the degree of underlying immune dysregulation in severe cases.

Skin biopsy is indicated if the diagnosis is in doubt.

Patch testing may be needed if there is coexistent contact dermatitis in order to help identify the offending antigen. Local application of house dust mite allergen has been used in research applications to demonstrate contact hypersensitivity in cases where it is considered a potential factor in worsening the condition.

Management

General comments

Eczema has substantial psychosocial consequences in addition to its disabling physical symptoms. There is a cultural aversion to skin diseases, born partly of fear of contagion and partly from appearances. This can have a serious effect on young people for whom peer acceptance is an important part of life. The itching and discomfort leads to sleep deprivation which in turn produces psychological problems. It is important, therefore, to establish a good relationship between patient and doctor. Patients often want 'a cause' to be found which when removed will lead to recovery, and the chronicity of the condition leads to great frustration in both patients and their doctors. It needs careful and repeated discussion to get the message across to patients that the disease is multifactorial and that attention to many aspects simultaneously is important for adequate control. Eczema can be treated as an outpatient in most circumstances but hospital admission may be necessary for intensive treatment to induce a remission in severe disease.

General measures

Avoid hot showers and baths—always use tepid water. Baths are preferable to showers so that patients can soak. Emulsified oatmeal and oily preparations are useful as antipruritic and moisturising agents. Use of soaps should be minimised and non-perfumed cleansing bars, such as Dermaveen, QV or

Pinetarsol, are preferable. Rubbing dry should be avoided and the use of a soft towel to pat dry is preferable.

Cotton gloves with barrier gloves over them should be worn when working with detergents or household cleaners.

Cotton instead of synthetic fabrics should be selected for underclothes and general clothing. Fingernails should be kept short and if necessary gloves worn at night to prevent scratching.

Factors responsible for generating emotional stress should be explored and confronted and psychological counselling may be necessary.

The opportunity may exist for providing advice regarding selection of the most appropriate careers. Less desirable are occupations which involve work in hot, dry or dusty conditions or work in wet environments, where frequent hand washing is required, rubber gloves need to be worn on a prolonged basis or high stress levels are encountered. Occupations with high levels of exposure to allergens such as work with laboratory animals or veterinary work should be avoided.

Topical therapy

This is the foundation of adequate management and must be continued irrespective of other forms of treatment. Creams are easier to use but less moisturising than ointments. Some commercially available preparations include lanolin and should be avoided in those patients who are lanolin-sensitive.

1. *For bathing and showering.* There are various bath oils and moisturisers which can be added to the bath for soaking or applied directly to the skin under a shower. They can be very soothing and remove the itching. They include preparations based on oatmeal, pine tar, liquid paraffin or dimethicone.

2. *Moisturisers.* These are essential on a regular daily basis, and after showering or bathing. They include sorbolene with glycerine, urea-based preparations and emulsifying ointments which are messy but effective. Urea increases absorption of other ingredients such as hydrocortisone, and so the combination should not be used on the face.

3. *Topical corticosteroids.* These are the mainstay of treatment. They are available as ointments or creams, the former more indicated with dry lesions. Preparations are classified on the basis of their potency. If used excessively, especially the more potent preparations, topical corticosteroids can lead to thinning of the skin and decreased collagen synthesis, resulting in a shiny, erythematous appearance with telangiectasia, striae and steroid purpura. The only topical steroids suitable for use on the face are hydrocortisone preparations in Class I, and mometasone and methylprednisolone aceponate which, despite their potency being equivalent to betamethasone diproprionate, have been claimed to be safe in children and on the face. In the presence of infection topical steroids can lead to aggravation of the condition. Used in high doses and especially when under occlusive dressings, topical steroids are absorbed in sufficient amounts to cause systemic effects.

Treatment of infection

The presence of crusting and weeping lesions, and especially pustules, indicates that there is bacterial infection, usually with *Staphylococcus aureus*, and a course of oral antibiotics such as flucloxacillin, cephalosporin or erythromycin is required to bring the eczema under control. Topical antibiotics are generally ineffective. Concomitant use of erythromycin and terfenadine or astemizole is contra-indicated.

Dietary management

Food hypersensitivity reactions can be a factor in eczema, especially in children. A trial of a hypo-allergenic diet is always worthwhile and this is usually based at least in part on the results of allergy investigations. In adults it is less common to find that specific allergic responses can be demonstrated but patients may notice some improvement when preservatives, colouring agents and other additives are removed from the diet. Sodium

TABLE 14.3 Topical corticosteroids for use on the skin

Potency	Preparations	Trade names
Class I Weak	Hydrocortisone 0.5–1%	Dermacort Squibb HC Egocort Sigmacort Cortef, Adacor
Class II Moderate	Alclometasone diproprionate 0.05%	Logoderm
	Betamethasone valerate 0.02%	Betnovate 1/5 cream Celestone M
	Betamethasone valerate 0.05%	Betnovate 1/2 Celestone V 1/2
	Triamcinolone acetonide, 0.02% and 0.05%	Aristocort Kenalone
	Fluocortolone pivalate/hexanoate 0.1%	Ultralan
Class III Strong	Betamethasone valerate 0.1%	Betnovate Celestone V
	Betamethasone diproprionate 0.05%	Diprosone Eleuphrat
	Mometasone furoate 0.1%	Elocon
	Methylprednisolone aceponate 0.1%	Advantan
	Triamcinolone acetonide 0.1%	Kenacomb*
	Fluclorolone acetonide 0.025%	Topilar
Class IV Very strong	Betamethasone diproprionate 0.5% Halcinonide 0.1%	Diprosone OV Halciderm

*Some preparations are combined with antimicrobial agents such as antibiotics, e.g. Kenacomb, Aristocomb, or clioquinol e.g. Vioform-Hydrocortisone.
(Adapted from 'A Current Therapeutics Guide, Topical Corticosteroids', Adis International Pty Ltd, Sydney, 1992 and 'New Ethicals Compendium', Adis International, Auckland, 1992).

cromoglycate by oral administration has been used where food allergy has been demonstrated but this agent is no longer available for this purpose in Australia. The doses required far exceed the formulations available for respiratory allergy, making it impractical to adapt the respiratory preparations for oral use.

Other agents

Antihistamines are useful for relieving the pruritus, especially at night. This helps to break the cycle of itching leading to scratching or rubbing of the skin resulting in lichenification, which in turn produces more itching. The older sedating antihistamines are effective and it is difficult to dissect out the sedative from the antihistamine properties. Publications have indicated efficacy with second generation antihistamines such as terfenadine and cetirizine. Hydroxyzine, which has some anxiolytic properties, is particularly valuable in eczema. A small nocturnal dose of doxepin is another effective agent and its soporific properties are useful.

Evening primrose oil has been claimed to be effective in eczema but the effects are usually only marginal and at least three months' trial is needed to gauge response. It is harmless but expensive.

Systemic corticosteroids are very effective in relieving the allergic inflammation and allowing healing of the eczematous lesions. However, the condition usually relapses promptly when the dosage is reduced. Oral steroids should not be used unless there are compelling reasons to do so.

Immunosuppressive agents. Cyclosporine has been used in severe eczema but it has significant drawbacks in the development of renal disease and predisposition to lymphoma. However, azathioprine has similar beneficial effects, and is an easier drug to use with less dramatic side effects. Both agents should be contemplated only in serious cases as part of specialist treatment.

Gamma interferon has been tried in severe atopic eczema with encouraging results. The rationale for its use is to switch T cell function from the Th2 to the Th1 profile.

Prognosis

Eczema in infants goes into remission in many cases. In adults and children where it accompanies other allergic diseases such as asthma and hayfever, it often behaves in a counter-cyclical fashion, remitting when respiratory symptoms are more prominent and worsening when they improve.

Poor prognostic indicators are the presence of severe disease, where extensor rather than flexor surfaces are involved, older age of onset and associated respiratory allergic disease.

When to refer patient to specialist

1. Where extensive disease or intense symptoms are interfering with sleep patterns and activities of daily living.

2. Where a food allergy is suspected. This is difficult to investigate and requires specialised knowledge, especially in children where overzealous adherence to diets can have potentially dangerous consequences.
3. Where the patient is distressed.
4. For the overall investigation of allergic factors, especially where there is a significant respiratory allergy component.

Background

Functional anatomy of the skin

The skin is a major organ system of the body, with many different functions which include forming a barrier to infection and foreign substances, supporting immune function by antigen presentation, fulfilling homeostatic and metabolic functions by maintaining an even temperature and conserving water and manufacturing Vitamin D, and acting as a sensory organ. It consists of epidermis, or outer layer, which in turn is composed of several layers. The outer corneum stratum is impervious to water and acts as a barrier. Cells are generated in the basal layer and migrate towards the stratum corneum from where they are shed. Water is retained in the middle layers of the epidermis and contributes to the suppleness of the skin. The skin becomes hard and brittle when dehydrated. Melanocytes are present in the basal layers of the skin and produce melanin pigment in response to sunlight, thereby protecting the skin from actinic radiation. The basal cells of the epidermis are located on the basement membrane. The dermis is situated beneath the basement membrane and consists of connective tissue which supports a rich blood supply system and numerous nerve endings. Within the dermis are sebaceous and sweat glands which provide the secretions which contribute to the integrity of the skin and assist in its various functions. Subcutaneous tissue beneath the dermis contains fat cells which act as insulators, energy storage and endocrine organ.

In eczema there are inflammatory changes through all levels of the skin. The epidermis shows hyperkeratosis, parakeratosis, spongiosis and oedema. In the dermis there is a perivascular infiltrate of mononuclear cells consisting of lymphocytes, monocytes and macrophages, and some inflammatory cells are also seen in the epidermis. Most of the lymphocytes are CD4+ T cells and are also HLA DR+ indicating activation. Eosinophils may also be prominent, especially in a flare after exposure to allergen.

Immunology of the skin

The skin is a major barrier between the internal environment and the external world and its allergens. It therefore fulfils important immunological roles in limiting access to antigen and in facilitating the interaction of the immune response with external antigens.

Between the epidermal cells are Langerhans cells. These are dendritic cells which form part of the system of antigen presenting cells throughout the body. They have long processes which facilitate contact with antigen. Once antigen is captured on their surfaces, Langerhans cells migrate through the afferent lymphatics to the regional lymph nodes where they present the antigen to T cells, together with MHC Class II molecules. They also have on their surfaces high affinity receptors for IgE ($Fc_\varepsilon RI$), which has major implications for function of these cells in relation to allergic diseases. Langerhans cells are highly susceptible to UV irradiation which reduces their numbers and function, resulting in significant immunosuppression.

Lymphocytes, mainly T cells, are scattered throughout the dermis, and some are present in the epidermis. In some areas they form aggregates. Macrophages in the dermis play a role in antigen processing.

Mast cells are present in the dermis and subcutaneous tissues where

FIGURE 14.2 **Schematic representation of mechanisms involved in the pathogenesis of eczema.**

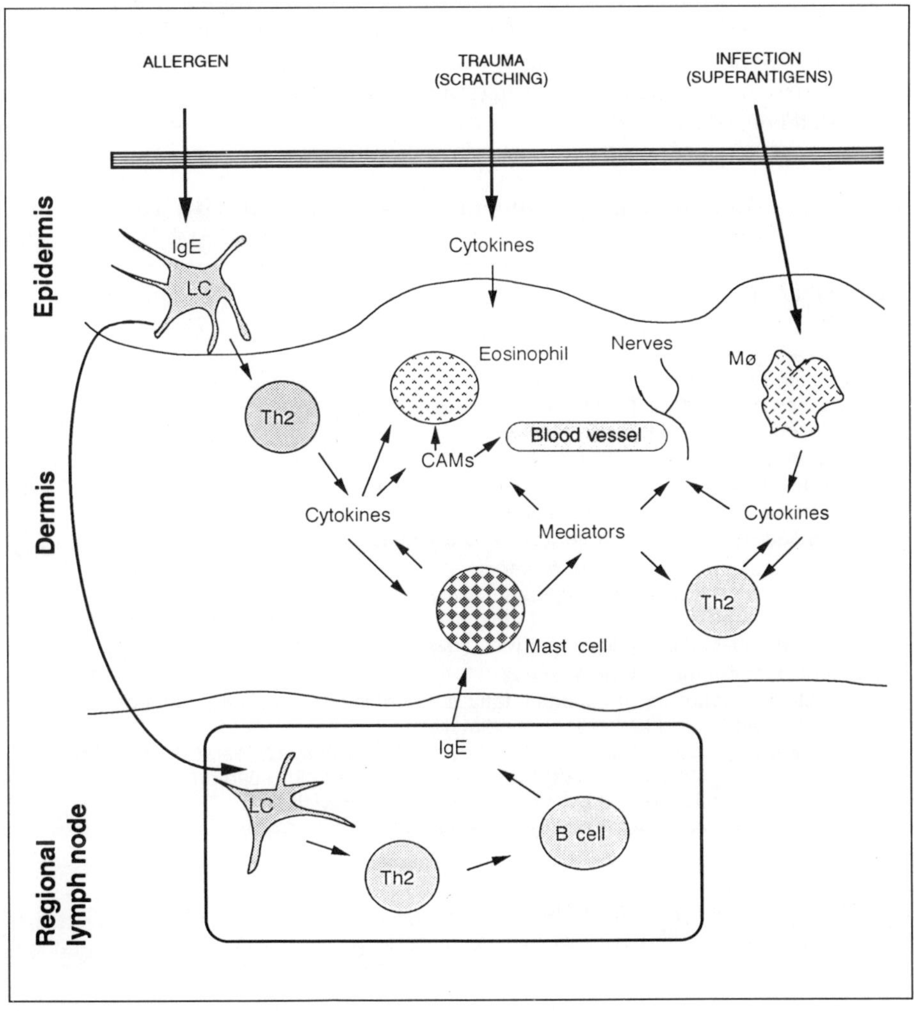

they are in close association with small nerve endings, providing substance to the interaction between the nervous and immune systems. Small numbers of eosinophils are present in the dermis. Their numbers are greatly increased in eczema and in inflammatory allergic reactions.

Pathophysiology of eczema

There is increasing evidence that the CD4+ helper cell profile in patients with atopy in general, and with atopic eczema in particular, is predominantly of the Th2 type. The cytokine profile of this population encourages production of IgE and recruitment of eosinophils. More recently another mechanism has been postulated in atopic eczema involving superantigens from the bacterial toxins of *Staphylococcus aureus* which colonises the skin of these patients. Superantigens are capable of inducing massive proliferation of certain restricted classes of T cells which favour allergic inflammation.

A number of disturbances in immunological function are present in atopic eczema, which can be explained by the altered cytokine profile consistent with the predominance of Th2 cells. There is impairment of cell-mediated immune function, overactivity of B cell function, especially IgE mechanisms, and disturbances of autonomic function and mediator release from mast cells have also been described.

TABLE 14.4 **Immunological abnormalities associated with atopic eczema**

Langerhans cells
T cells
Circulating T cell lymphopenia
Increased CD4:8 ratio
Reduced numbers of T cells in skin
Reduced responsiveness to mitogens ConA and PHA
B cells
High IgE levels
Association with other atopic diseases
Immediate hypersensitivity reactions to a variety of environmental allergens
Functional cell-mediated immune defects
Hypoergy on delayed type hypersensitivity skin tests
Reduced sensitisation to contact antigens such as dinitrochlorobenzene (DNCB)
Increased susceptibility to fungal (candidal) and viral infections
Mediator release and responsiveness
Defective metabolism of essential fatty acids which are the precursors of prostaglandin and leukotriene mediators
Decreased cyclic AMP and increased cyclic AMP phosphodiesterase resulting in abnormal signal transduction from α and β adrenergic receptors
Abnormal vascular responses to histamine and acetylcholine
Association with immunodeficiency diseases
Wiskott-Aldrich syndrome
Ataxia-telangiectasia
X-linked agammaglobulinaemia
Hyper-IgE syndrome

Mechanism of action of therapeutic interventions

Our better understanding of the pathogenesis of eczema has therapeutic implications. Trials with IFN-γ, which down-regulate Th2 cells, have shown some clinical benefit. Reduced T cell function by use of cyclosporine and azathioprine has proved useful in some cases. The superantigen story gives credence to the clinical observation of improvement with prolonged courses of antistaphylococcal antibiotics. The beneficial effect sometimes observed of gamolenic acid administration in evening primrose oil may be explained by its effects on the metabolism of leukotrienes and prostaglandins.

Further reading

Hunter JAA, Herd RM. Recent advances in atopic dermatitis. *Quart J Med* 1994; 87: 323–7.

Leung DYM. Atopic dermatitis: the skin as a window into the pathogenesis of chronic allergic diseases. *J Allergy Clin Immunol* 1995; 96: 302–18.

Williams HC, Burney PGJ, Pembroke AC, Hay RJ. The UK Working Party's diagnostic criteria for atopic dermatitis III: independent hospital evaluation. *Br J Dermatol* 1994; 131: 406–16.

Chapter 15

Urticaria and angioedema

Urticaria is a common condition. In its chronic form it is one of the most frustrating conditions seen in clinical practice, both for patients and their doctors.

Definition

Urticaria, also known as hives, is characterised by transient, pruritic, oedematous wheals or erythematous papules. The important features which distinguish it from other skin conditions are its transient nature and its intense burning itch. Individual lesions last no longer than 24 hours and disappear without leaving any sequelae, to be followed by others in a dynamic waxing and waning of different lesions.

Angioedema is a condition with transient swelling of deeper dermal and subcutaneous tissues, thought to be of similar pathogenesis to urticaria. In about half the cases of urticaria there is associated angioedema which makes the prognosis worse.

Classification

Urticaria and angioedema can be classified on the basis of:

1. *The duration of symptoms.* This is an important distinction because acute and chronic urticaria differ considerably in several respects. Acute urticaria is arbitrarily defined as lasting less than 6 weeks. It occurs predominantly in atopic subjects, and hence is seen most commonly in children. Both sexes are equally affected. Its onset can often be related to a particular allergen or to a viral infection. Probably many patients do not consult a doctor.

   Chronic urticaria refers to disease persisting on a continuous or intermittent basis for more than 6 weeks. It is more common in middle life, and more women than men are affected. There is no greater frequency in patients with atopy and the cause is often difficult to establish.

2. *Whether the two conditions occur together.* The presence of angioedema makes the prognosis worse and the condition tends to persist longer.

3. *Pathogenesis.* This has important implications for therapy and prognosis.

   (a) Idiopathic. No cause can be found. This is the commonest form of chronic urticaria.

(b) Food related.

(c) Physical urticarias, such as cold induced, pressure or cholinergic urticaria.

(d) Associated with underlying disease.

(e) Hereditary.

Clinical features

Urticaria is intensely itchy. It is pleomorphic, varying in size from a few millimetres to several centimetres, and of any shape. Individual lesions persist for less than 12 to 24 hours, and in most cases less than 4 hours. New lesions may appear in crops or more or less continuously. They leave no marks when they disappear. Distribution of the lesions is widespread and of little aetiological significance except in special situations such as contact urticaria where the lesions appear at the site of contact with the precipitating factor, solar urticaria which occurs in the sun-exposed areas, and some other physical urticarias such as pressure urticaria which are localised to sites where the stimulus is applied.

There are no associated systemic symptoms but the patient may feel hot if the lesions are severe and widespread. There may be joint symptoms from proximity of lesions to joints, but polyarthralgia should raise suspicion of an underlying disease.

Angioedema may produce no discomfort if in loose tissue, but is frequently heralded by a stinging, burning sensation. Angioedema in restricted areas can produce pain, obstruction to airways and hoarseness; in bowel wall it produces abdominal cramps, diarrhoea and vomiting (visceral involvement is particularly likely with hereditary angioedema); adjacent to joints it may produce arthralgia. Acute urticaria and angioedema can be associated with hypotension and bronchospasm and form part of the syndrome of anaphylaxis.

Urticaria should be regarded as a syndrome rather than a disease, implying that it is important to look for an underlying cause in all cases. Features which suggest the presence of underlying disease are the presence of constitutional symptoms such as fatigue, weight loss, fever and the presence of arthralgia or arthritis. A full history and examination is necessary in all cases to ensure that there are no indications of underlying disease such as lymphadenopathy or signs of thyrotoxicosis.

An *underlying vasculitis* should be suspected when individual lesions last longer than 24 hours, there is brownish discolouration, scarring or induration in the sites of previous wheals, if palpable purpura is present and with preferential involvement of lower limbs.

Pruritic urticarial papules and plaques of pregnancy (PUPPP) is an intensely itchy condition which affects predominantly primigravidae in the third trimester of pregnancy. It usually subsides in the postpartum period. It is of unknown aetiology. The common variety of chronic idiopathic urticaria also occurs in pregnancy, which can lead to worsening or improvement of the condition.

Physical urticarias

Certain forms of urticaria have characteristic appearances, notably the physical urticarias. They account for between 7 and 17% of cases of chronic urticaria. They are usually short-lived and confined to the area of application of the stimulus. Some of their characteristics can, however, accompany chronic idiopathic urticaria. For example, it is not uncommon to find that urticarial wheals are more abundant under tight clothing.

Cold urticaria is by far the most important of the physical urticarias since the potential exists for massive mediator release with bronchospasm and syncope, and it can be a factor in deaths from drowning. Serum levels of histamine and other mediators are elevated. Underlying diseases producing cryoglobulinaemia, connective tissue and lymphoproliferative diseases need to be excluded. The ice-cube test is positive in a high proportion of patients. An ice-cube is enclosed in a water-tight covering and applied to the skin for 5 minutes. The development of a wheal in the area of application constitutes a positive result.

Dermatographism is demonstrated by stroking the skin with a blunt object such as a pen or the finger. A wheal is produced in the area of pressure. This may be the predominant symptom or it may accompany many other forms of urticaria.

Delayed pressure urticaria occurs 3 to 12 hours after local application of pressure such as after carrying a shoulder bag. This is a refractory, steroid-dependent condition.

Cholinergic urticaria consists of characteristic small (2–3 mm) wheals with large erythematous flares. It is precipitated by warmth, emotional stress and exercise. Intradermal injection of methacholine reproduces the lesions in about 50% of patients.

Solar urticaria is limited to sun-exposed areas and may be accompanied by wheezing, dizziness, headache and collapse after prolonged exposure. It is classified according to the inciting wavelength of light and can be passively transferred with serum.

Aquagenic urticaria is a rare form of urticaria precipitated by exposure of the skin to water, irrespective of its temperature. Its appearance is similar to that of cholinergic urticaria.

Exercise-induced urticaria and angioedema. This can form part of the syndrome of anaphylaxis. Elevated serum histamine levels are found. Sometimes the syndrome is reproduced only when exercise is undertaken after ingestion of certain foods, especially wheat products.

Diagnosis

The diagnosis of urticaria and angioedema is usually obvious from the clinical picture and the history. However, it is important to establish whether there is an underlying cause for the condition. Investigations in chronic urticaria are often negative, but if none are undertaken and patients are treated symptomatically without explanation they are unlikely to be satisfied and will seek another opinion. It is important to explain the syndrome and the expectations of finding a cause. The causes of urticaria and angioedema differ in acute and chronic urticaria.

Acute urticaria

Drug reactions are among the most commonly recognised causes, with penicillin being the commonest drug implicated. Dermatographism may persist for months after the acute reaction has settled. The role of traces of penicillin in foodstuffs, predominantly dairy products, in producing chronic urticaria, is unproved. ACE inhibitors have become a common cause of angioedema without urticaria.

Foods are frequently involved and are readily identified. The response is usually mediated through IgE. Frequent offenders are peanuts, nuts, fish, shellfish, eggs, milk, chocolate, tomatoes and fresh berries. Particularly violent reactions are liable to occur with very small amounts of peanuts, nuts, fish, legumes and eggs. The variability in reaction may be explained by such factors as dosage, presentation, cooking and factors altering rates of absorption. Lobster, crayfish, egg white, mussels and strawberries may act as pharmacological histamine releasing agents.

Inhalant allergens in most cases cause respiratory symptoms at the same time as the urticaria. Animal danders including laboratory animals are the most common offending agents.

Infections. Acute viral infections are a common cause of acute urticaria, especially in children. Usually the virus is not isolated, but it can be associated with identified viruses, including hepatitis B (less frequently hepatitis A), infectious mononucleosis and Coxsackie. Streptococcal pharyngitis in children may occasionally be associated with urticaria.

Chronic urticaria

Drugs also need to be considered in chronic urticaria, even if there has been no recent change in drug intake. It is important to ask about non-prescription items as well as prescribed drugs. From 20 to 40% of patients with chronic urticaria will find that their symptoms worsen with aspirin, and many react to non-steroidal anti-inflammatory agents (NSAIDs) suggesting a pharmacological effect through inhibition of cyclo-oxygenase. Aspirin-sensitive patients also react to tartrazine and benzoates. The reaction may be caused not by the active ingredient of the medication but by colouring agents or other constituents of the formulation. Substitution of white tablets for multicoloured capsules can sometimes solve the problem.

Foods. The role of foodstuffs in causing chronic urticaria is controversial, and the reported prevalence ranges from 1% to 67%. Part of this discrepancy is accounted for by the vigour with which this possibility is pursued. However, the number of patients in whom food can be incriminated has diminished over the past decade, possibly because of increased awareness of preservatives, colouring agents and other additives in foods. In chronic urticaria foods cause reactions predominantly through the pharmacological effects of additives and preservatives, and IgE mechanisms are not involved.

Infections. Focal infection, especially sinus, dental and tonsillar were at one time believed to be important causes of urticaria. Although the association is difficult to prove it is worth searching for occult infection in the refractory, severe case when other causes have been excluded.

Fungal infection. There is a recent vogue for ascribing angioedema and urticaria to occult candidiasis, and claims have been made for oral antifungal agents and low yeast diets, especially by complementary (alternative) medicine practitioners. There is no good evidence to support this association. Other fungal infections have also been incriminated, including tinea pedis with anecdotal reports of improvement in urticaria when the infection is dealt with.

Parasites should be suspected if a marked eosinophilia and very high serum IgE are found. However, this is very rarely a problem in Australia, and routine stool testing for cysts, ova and parasites is not justified.

Contactants can produce generalised urticaria and even anaphylaxis through absorption on occasions. This has been reported mainly in response to antibiotics, especially ampicillin, bacitracin, neomycin, penicillin, streptomycin and chloramphenicol, insect repellants and sunscreen preparations, but it has also been described with egg, balsam of Peru and epoxy resins.

Underlying disease must be considered in any patient who presents with urticaria, particularly if there are systemic features such as fever or weight loss, or if it develops for the first time in older age. Although unusual, urticaria may be the presenting feature of some systemic diseases or develop at some stage during their course. This association has been reported with:

(a) *autoimmune diseases*, including SLE which may present with urticaria in about 8% of cases, juvenile rheumatoid arthritis, rheumatic fever, necrotizing vasculitis and polymyositis;

(b) *endocrine disorders*, especially thyroid autoimmunity, including thyrotoxicosis. Urticaria is often worse in the premenstrual period and has been associated with pregnancy;

(c) *malignant disease*, and there are reports of clearing with resection of the tumour in some cases. Acquired C1-inhibitor deficiency has been described with lymphomas and carcinomas, and these patients respond to antifibrinolytic and androgen therapy in the same way as do patients with hereditary angioedema (HAE);

(d) *inherited disorders.* With the exception of C3b-inactivator deficiency (recessive), all are autosomal dominant disorders. They are very rare diseases, except for *hereditary angioedema*, due to deficiency of the inhibitor of the first component of complement, C1q (C1INH). In 15% of kindred the protein is measurable by immunochemical techniques but is not functional. A macular erythematous rash may precede episodes of angioedema, but there is no urticaria. Mortality from respiratory obstruction occurred in 20–30% of subjects before modern therapy. HAE accounts for about 2% of all cases of angioedema. Pathogenesis was ascribed to C2 kinin, a split product of C2 from continued activation of complement pathways, but more recent studies suggest spontaneous generation of bradykinin.

Investigations

Careful history and physical examination may provide clues to possible underlying causes such as the relationship to food, recent viral illness or the presence of connective tissue disease. Characteristic features of specific syndromes may be apparent, for example cholinergic urticaria, dermatographism, or urticaria pigmentosa. In most cases, however, there are no clues to the diagnosis.

Where clinical features suggest another disease is present which may be relevant to the development of urticaria, the appropriate laboratory investigations are undertaken. However, where there are no clues to possible aetiology and where the clinical picture is one of uncomplicated urticaria and angioedema, there is diversity of opinion regarding the value of laboratory investigations. Up to 20% of such patients have been found to have abnormal laboratory results but this does not necessarily translate into clinically meaningful information. 'Routine' testing has a low yield. Examination of stools for parasites is nearly always fruitless and should not be performed without good reason. If vasculitis is suspected, it is necessary to biopsy one of the lesions for examination by conventional light microscopy, as well as immunofluorescence. Serum complement estimations and antinuclear antibody should also be done. Sinus and dental X-rays have been reported to be positive in up to 17% of cases with improvement of urticaria following appropriate treatment.

Skin prick tests are helpful in acute urticaria for identifying potential allergens such as insect stings and foods, but they are of little value in patients with chronic urticaria. These patients are frequently not atopic and specific IgE mechanisms are seldom involved.

Physical urticarias can be demonstrated using a number of specific manoeuvres to provoke a reaction. These include stroking of skin in dermatographism, application of an ice-cube to the skin in cold urticaria, exposure to specific wavelengths of light in solar urticaria, and exercise in cholinergic and exercise-induced urticaria.

A proportion of patients with chronic idiopathic urticaria have intolerance to various food additives which may not be apparent from the clinical presentation. Although the proportion of these patients appears to be far less now than previously, it is still worthwhile considering food intolerance. Serial exclusion of suspected foods is unlikely to be successful and the only reliable investigation is a formal elimination diet, maintained for 2 weeks while a diary is kept of foods and symptoms over the period. If the patient becomes asymptomatic, it is likely that a food reaction is present. There are now two possible routes to follow. Capsules containing various food chemicals or placebos are taken, one on each successive day so that the patient is unaware of their contents. At the end of the process the code is broken and any reactions can be identified. The other possibility is to perform an open challenge by adding foods back to the diet every 48 hours. Any suspected reaction can be confirmed later by blinded challenge with the suspected food. Further details are provided in Chapter 17.

Psychological factors contribute frequently to the syndrome and need to be identified by enquiring specifically into these aspects of the illness. Formal psychological assessment and management may be required on occasions.

Differential diagnosis

Urticaria can be mistaken for several skin disorders which are itchy or have bullae or papules. These include:

(a) *urticarial vasculitis*, often difficult to distinguish from idiopathic chronic urticaria. Lesions tend to be less transient and may leave brown staining of the skin when they subside. Urticarial vasculitis is one pole of a spectrum of conditions which at the other extreme has the features of systemic lupus erythematosus with vasculitis. There is hypocomplementaemia and a positive antinuclear antibody. Skin biopsy should be performed on a high index of suspicion and will show vasculitic changes with deposition of immunoglobulin and complement in basement membrane and blood vessels.

(b) *erythema multiforme.* There is a spectrum of appearances from urticarial lesions through variable erythema including target lesions, to bullae. Lesions are relatively fixed, tend to burn or sting rather than itch, and there may be a prodromal illness or constitutional symptoms. The conditions can be distinguished histologically. In the severe form of erythema multiforme there is high fever and mucosal involvement. The condition is precipitated by a number of factors, particularly drugs, infections and malignancy.

(c) *papular urticaria*, which consists of itchy, persistent papules, usually on the lower limbs, and represents a hypersensitivity reaction to insect bites.

(d) *bullous pemphigoid*, especially in the early stages, can have an urticarial component. This usually occurs in older patients. About 70% of patients will have circulating auto-antibody with specificity for basement membrane. Skin biopsy shows deposition of immunoglobulin and complement in the basement membrane where cleavage of skin occurs.

(e) *dermatitis herpetiformis* may also show isolated intensely itchy bullous lesions, predominantly around knees, elbows, buttocks, sacral and shoulder areas. It is associated with gluten intolerance.

(f) *urticaria pigmentosa*, which may be part of systemic mastocytosis, has persistent, papular pigmented lesions. Stroking of the skin overlying the lesions produces a linear urticarial wheal known as Darier's sign. Diagnosis is confirmed by skin biopsy which on special staining shows clusters of mast cells.

Management

1. The disease should be explained to the patient. If this is not done, and no attempts are made to find an underlying cause, patients become frustrated and gravitate to other practitioners, especially in chronic cases.
2. Find and remove the cause. Food intolerance, psychological factors, and underlying disease must be considered. In most cases no identifiable

cause can be found, and then treatment is necessary to suppress symptoms.

3. Suppress the symptoms. Antihistamines are the mainstay of treatment. The advent of non-sedating or low-sedating drugs has led to a significant improvement in quality of life for these patients. Often the dosage needs to be higher than for other indications and the medication needs to be given on a regular basis rather than as required. Antihistamines displace histamine from its receptors and they are more effective if given prior to the onset of symptoms and continued on a regular basis. Concern about cardiac toxicity of some of these drugs such as terfenadine and astemizole have put a stop to the practice of titrating the dose upwards until an effect is obtained, while with other drugs such as loratadine and cetirizine, increasing the dose may lead to sedation. Hydroxyzine is a first generation antihistamine which is particularly effective in urticaria, possibly because of its tranquillising properties. Cetirizine is a derivative of this drug. If there is an imperfect response to one antihistamine, it is worth trying one of the others on its own or in combination. Doxepin, although indicated as an antidepressant, is also a powerful antihistamine. Some success has been claimed for its use in urticaria when other antihistamines have failed. Hydroxyzine and cyproheptadine are specifically indicated for cholinergic and cold urticaria respectively. However, sedation is a problem and non-sedating antihistamines are now used in the first instance in these conditions.

4. Options when antihistamines do not work:
   (a) Addition of an H2 antagonist such as cimetidine can bring the condition under control. H2 receptors are present in skin and blood vessels and play a pathogenetic role.
   (b) Adrenergic agents. It has been suggested that β-2 agonists such as terbutaline given orally may potentiate the effects of antihistamines, but they have not proved to be particularly effective.
   (c) Several agents have been reported to be useful in refractory urticaria. These include nifedipine, a calcium channel blocking agent; non-steroidal anti inflammatory agents (NSAIDs) such as indomethacin which are effective in urticarial vasculitis, but may be helpful also in some cases of chronic urticaria. However, they may exacerbate the condition in some patients through their 'aspirin-like' effects on cyclo-oxygenase pathways; dapsone controls symptoms in some cases of chronic refractory urticaria, especially if associated with vasculitis. However, its side effects limit its usefulness; danazol and tranexamic acid may be useful in some cases. Their primary use is in hereditary angioedema.

4. Corticosteroids are highly effective agents in urticaria and angioedema. After control is achieved with initial therapy of 40 to 60 mg per day, the dose should be reduced progressively to the lowest which will control symptoms. Side effects are reduced significantly if alternate day therapy can be achieved. Other than for life-saving indications they should be used only after other drugs have been tried.

Treatment of specific syndromes

Hereditary angioedema

Acute attacks do not respond to adrenaline, antihistamines or steroids. Fresh frozen plasma dramatically reverses the clinical picture, although the objection to its use is that it supplies not only the missing C1INH, but also the substrate for C1esterase, thereby having the potential for aggravating an attack. Purified C1INH preparations are now available.

Prophylaxis. Danazol, an attenuated androgen is particularly effective. It raises C1INH blood levels, but is effective even when normal levels are not achieved. It is also effective in variants with measurable but functionally inactive C1INH. It is contra-indicated in children and during pregnancy. Hepatotoxicity and virilising properties need to be considered. Tranexamic acid (cyclokapron), an antifibrinolytic agent and analogue of EACA (ε-amino caproic acid), is effective therapy. Side effects include thrombosis, but these are less common with tranexamic acid than with EACA.

Prognosis

It is difficult to predict the outcome of urticaria and angioedema. Acute urticaria in childhood is usually self-limited and will settle within a few weeks after recovery from an infection, or if the offending food is withdrawn. Many children have only one or a few such episodes and they do not recur. In most cases they also seem to be able to tolerate the offending foodstuff again later without difficulty.

There are few studies of the prognosis in chronic urticaria. Not surprisingly the prognosis is worse the longer the symptoms have been present, but there are few features of prognostic significance. If an underlying cause can be identified and removed, the prognosis is much better. In several studies in children and adults one to two thirds of cases resolve in the first few years, while up to half continue to have symptoms to a variable degree.

When to refer patient to specialist

Children with acute urticaria and especially where there is an obvious precipitating cause such as a food or a recent viral illness, usually run a self-limited course and need medication to suppress symptoms. However, patients who are proving refractory to treatment, or where there are features to suggest an underlying illness may need further investigation. Patients with life-threatening angioedema should be referred.

Background

Urticaria and angioedema have a cumulative prevalence in the general population of 15 to 25%. This means that one person in five experiences at least one episode of urticaria, angioedema or both during their lifetime.

Pathology

In acute urticaria there is oedema of the dermis, with dilatation of smaller cutaneous blood vessels, dilated lymphatics and a minimal perivascular infiltrate with mononuclear cells and eosinophils.

In chronic urticaria there is a more prominent perivascular infiltrate of mononuclear cells composed of T cells and macrophages. The presence of eosinophils is suggested by the presence of major basic protein. They are difficult to demonstrate with conventional light microscopy as most are degranulated and are seen only on electron microscopy. Mast cells are increased in numbers in the dermis and they show varying degrees of degranulation. Immunofluorescence studies of skin biopsies show no deposition of immunoglobulin, complement or fibrin.

When urticaria is associated with vasculitis there is necrosis of blood vessels and endothelial cell swelling of post capillary venules. The perivascular infiltrate consists predominantly of neutrophils which show leukocytoclasis, a term which indicates death of neutrophils with increased density of nuclei and nuclear fragments. There is extravasation of red blood cells and fibrinoid deposits are seen around venules. Immunofluorescence shows deposits of immunoglobulin (especially IgM), complement components and fibrin in vessel walls.

Pathogenesis

The central role of *mast cells* in this disease is supported by a number of findings. Increased numbers of mast cells are present in the lesions of chronic urticaria and there is evidence of their degranulation with increased release of histamine. Mediators released from mast cells have a number of biological effects which account for the clinical presentation of urticaria.

There are a number of mechanisms by which mast cells can be activated leading to their degranulation and release of mediators. These can be divided into immunological, non-immunological and dysfunctional interactions between IgE and its receptor.

Immunological mechanisms. IgE mediated reactions occur most commonly in acute urticaria. Curiously, IgE mechanisms also occur in some patients with cold and solar urticarias, and in dermographism, conditions where injection of IgE from a patient into the skin of another subject transfers the ability to react to the stimulus. Other mechanisms involve complement activation with generation of small fragments (C3a and C5a) which act as anaphylotoxins causing mast cell activation. This occurs in some drug reactions, collagen-vascular disorders, in patients with urticarial vasculitis and in transfusion reactions accompanied by urticaria.

Histamine releasing factors (HRF) induce histamine release from mast cells more rapidly than through IgE or other mechanisms. They are a heterogeneous group of molecules released from various activated cells, including monocytes/macrophages, platelets, lymphocytes, neutrophils and fibroblasts. Some HRF are generated as a result of IgE mechanisms. Mediator release can also be induced by a number of cytokines such as IL-3, IL-1 and GM-CSF released from various activated cells.

FIGURE 15.1 **Pathogenesis of urticaria.**

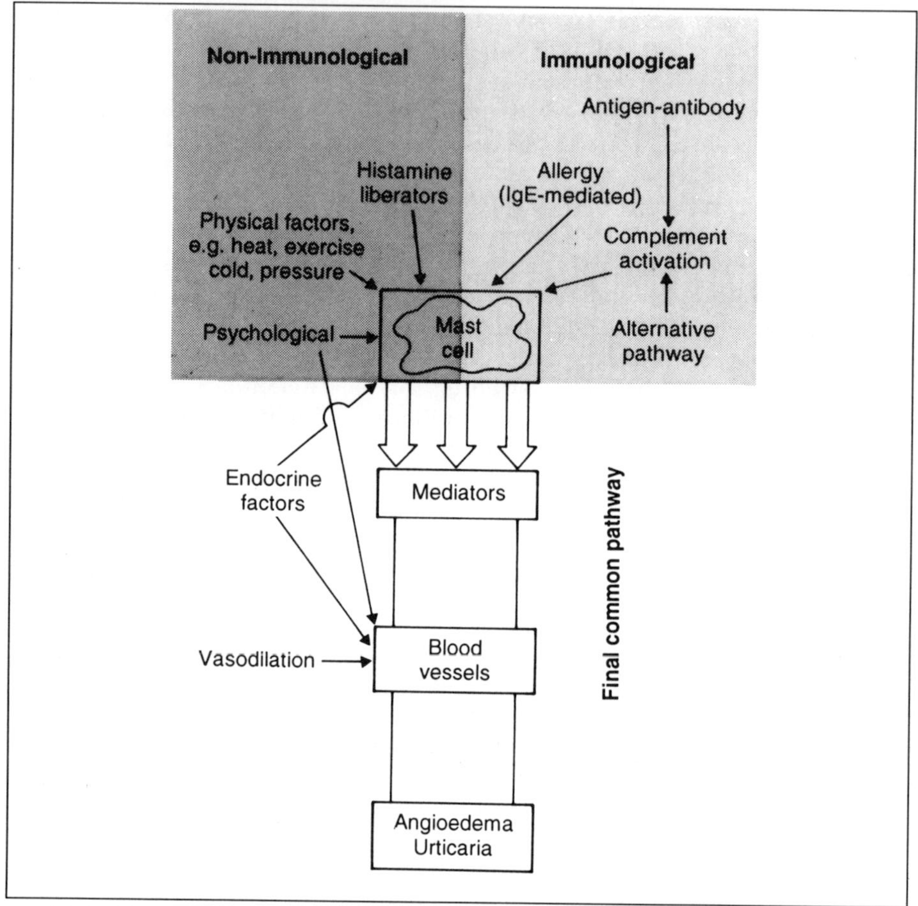

Reprinted with permission from Walls RS. Angioedema and urticaria. Common problems, uncommonly understood. Patient Management 1986;10:106–122.

Some patients with chronic urticaria have a serum factor which, when injected into their skin, induces a wheal and flare reaction. This has been shown to be an anti-IgE autoantibody. Later experiments demonstrated the presence of an autoantibody with specificity for the α sub-unit of the high affinity receptor for IgE (Fc$_\varepsilon$RI).

Non-immunological mechanisms of mediator release include direct histamine release by various drugs and foods such as morphine, codeine, meperidine, d-tubocurarine, polymyxin antibiotics, chlortetracycline, quinine, thiamine, aspirin, dextran, egg white, strawberries and a component of some shellfish and crustaceans. Physical stimuli such as stroking, pressure, heat and exercise can also induce mediator release.

The biochemical pathways within mast cells which lead to their degranulation and the secretion of mediators, is described in Chapter 26.

Histamine exerts its effects in the skin primarily through H1 and H2 receptors situated on blood vessels, resulting in vasodilatation and increased vascular permeability. It also stimulates sensory nerve endings, resulting in release of neuropeptides, including substance P, and in characteristically intense itching. Intradermal injection of histamine results in the triple wheal and flare response of Lewis which is analogous to the urticarial lesion. The wheal is due to increased vascular permeability and oedema, and the surrounding erythematous flare is due to vasodilatation and antidromic neuronal stimulation and release of substance P. H2 receptor stimulation results in increased production of certain interleukins which have an immunomodulatory effect. Activation of arachidonic acid pathways leads to release of prostaglandins, leukotrienes and platelet activating factor (PAF) which have important effects on vascular permeability and activation of other inflammatory cells. A variety of cytokines are also released with further important pro-inflammatory results.

The kinin pathway is activated by extravasation of plasma proteins and heparin release resulting from mast cell activity. Bradykinin is a potent vasoactive molecule which may be particularly important in development of angioedema.

End-organ reactivity

Various factors influence the responsiveness of blood vessels to histamine and other mediators. Increased responses to kallikrein and bradykinin have been noted in patients with chronic urticaria when compared to normal subjects. Hormonal effects also appear to influence responsiveness of blood vessels. It is common experience that women have worse symptoms in the premenstrual period. Auto-antibody to progesterone has been described but it is also likely that the steroids could have a modulating effect on responsiveness of blood vessels to mediators. Heat, alcohol and other vasodilators exacerbate urticaria through their vascular effects.

Further reading

1. Matthews KP. Urticaria and angioedema. Continuing medical education. *J Allergy Clin Immunol* 1983; 72: 1–14.
2. Charlesworth EN. The spectrum of urticaria. *In:* Charlesworth EN (ed). Immunology and Allergy Clinics of North America, 1995; 15: 641–57.

Algorithm: Approach to urticaria

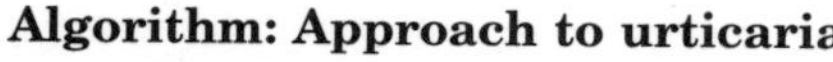

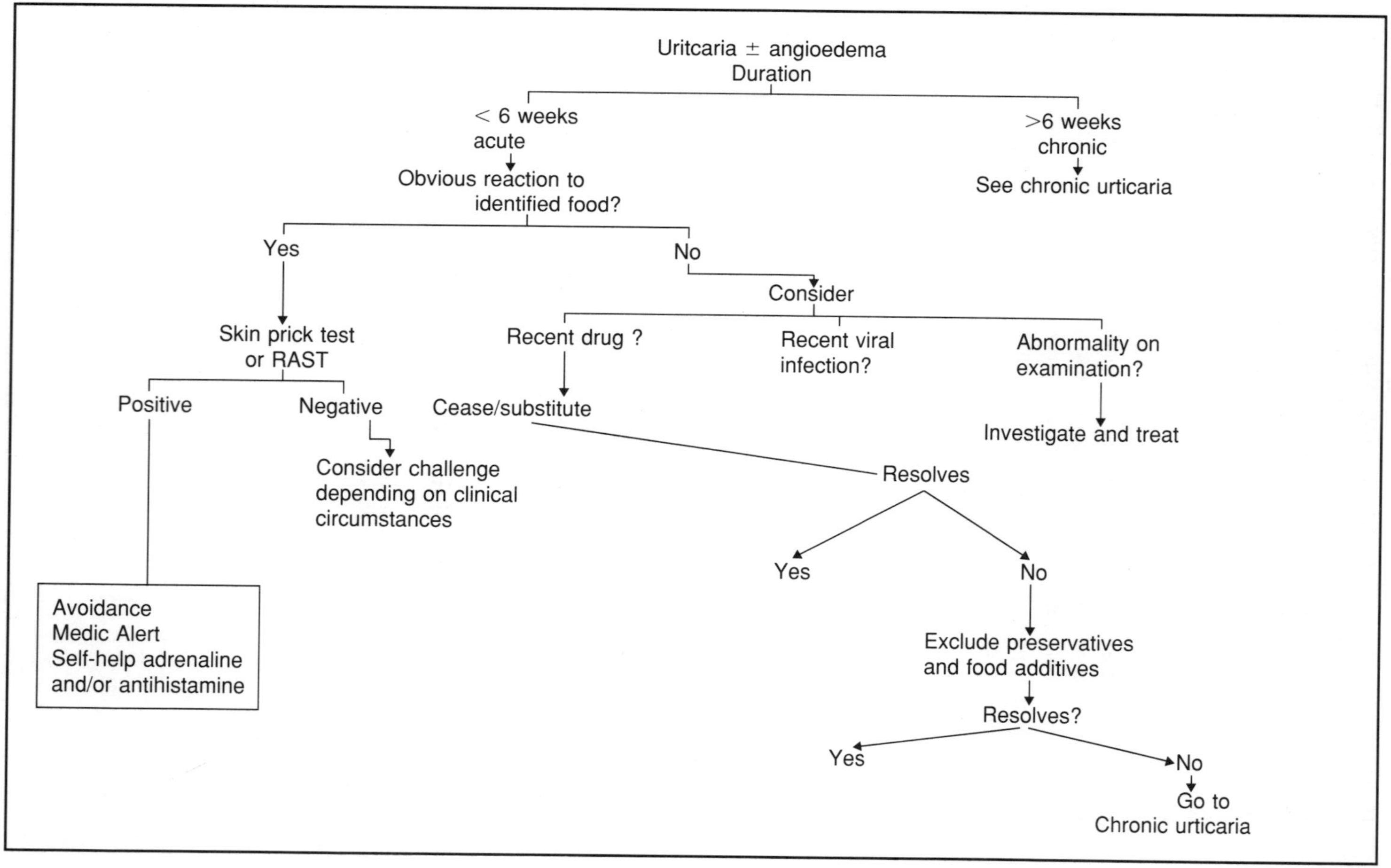

cont.

Algorithm: Approach to urticaria *cont*.

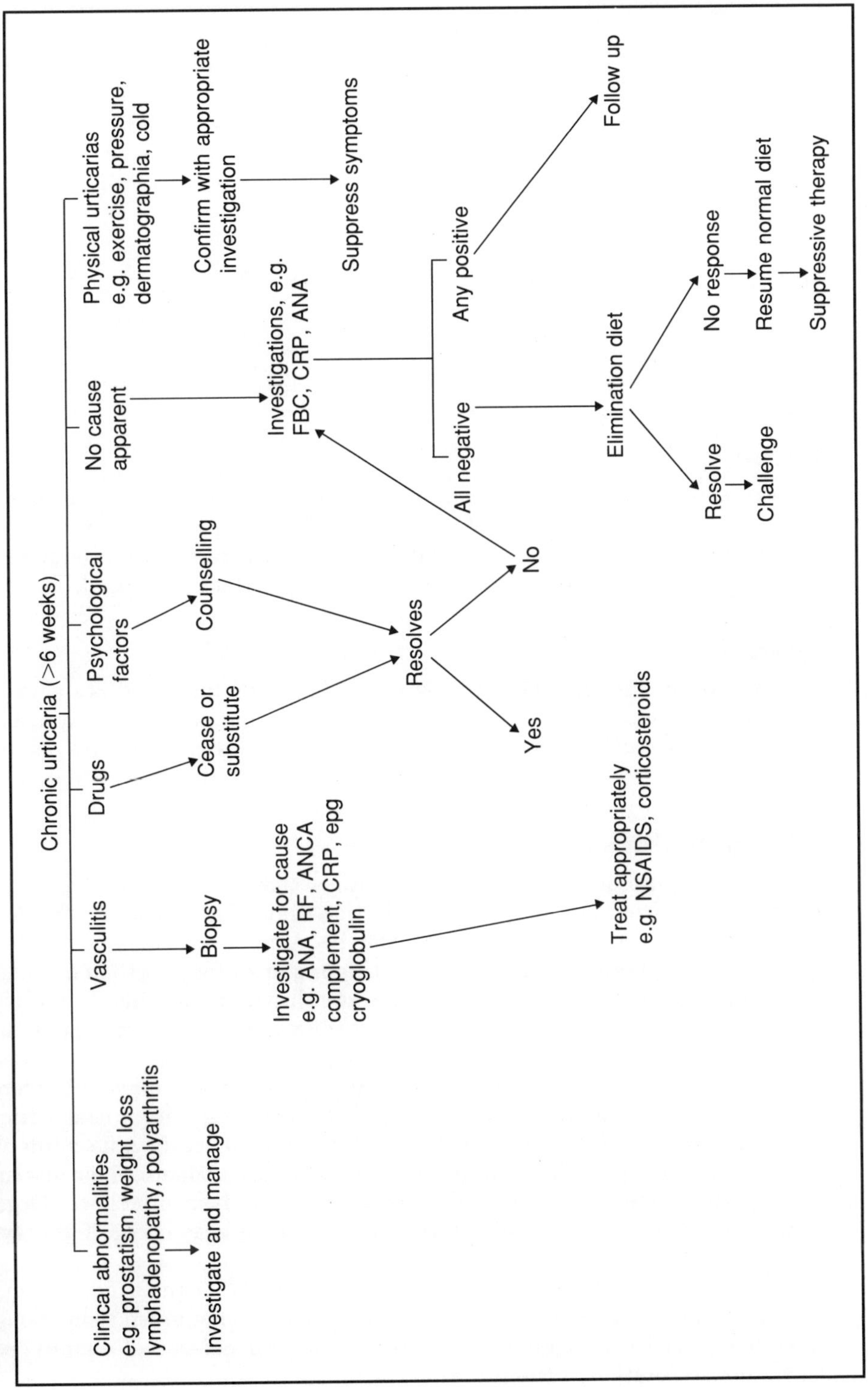

Chapter 16

Anaphylaxis

Introduction

Anaphylaxis is a generalised allergic reaction which results in a dramatic and usually unexpected medical emergency. The outcome is directly related to the speed of intervention. A similar clinical picture can be produced by mechanisms other than IgE, when the term anaphylactoid is used.

Definition

Anaphylaxis is the clinical manifestation of an IgE mediated response to allergen, expressed as a generalised reaction affecting primarily respiratory and cardiovascular systems, which if untreated results in shock and respiratory failure.

Clinical features

The onset of symptoms usually occurs within seconds or minutes of exposure to allergen. It is more rapid following injection than after ingestion. The more rapid the onset, the more severe it tends to be. Anaphylaxis may be heralded by restlessness, faintness, pruritus and tingling or diffuse erythema, coughing, change in voice, a feeling of a lump in the throat or sneezing. It develops rapidly into a syndrome involving the cardiovascular system, upper and lower respiratory system and skin. Tachycardia, hypotension and shock are due to hypovolaemia, and later cardiogenic shock may supervene. Angioedema involving the upper airways can cause respiratory obstruction, and there may also be intense bronchoconstriction. Urticaria causes intense itching and distress. The patient may experience abdominal or uterine cramps with a feeling of wanting to defaecate or of dysmenorrhoea. Organ damage including myocardial infarction and stroke may occur if the syndrome is not rapidly reversed.

Loss of consciousness and death can occur rapidly, or the syndrome may become refractory to treatment if adequate therapy is not given soon enough or is unsuccessful. In some patients, a second later episode of anaphylaxis may follow resolution of the initial event.

Diagnosis

A rapid history and examination are carried out while instituting resuscitation. The diagnosis is essentially clinical. Recent administration of a drug, some other well-defined precipitating event such as an insect sting, a history of previous episodes or of a specific allergy, all provide valuable clues to the diagnosis and the identity of the offending material. Identifiable risk factors for anaphylaxis include parenteral as opposed to oral administration of a drug, previous mild reactions to the same drug or stimulus, and concurrent treatment with β-blockers, drugs which are associated with severe anaphylaxis which is difficult to reverse. Where the diagnosis is in doubt, measurement of serum tryptase one to six hours after the onset of the episode can be diagnostic in retrospect.

An attempt should always be made to identify the precipitant of anaphylaxis in order to offer advice on avoiding future episodes. Skin prick testing with the suspected allergen will confirm the presence of specific IgE antibodies. This may be followed by intradermal testing in the case of insect sting and certain drug reactions. However, these procedures are hazardous where anaphylaxis has occurred and they should be undertaken only by practitioners experienced in provocation techniques and resuscitation.

Differential diagnosis

Sudden collapse may occur in the absence of urticaria and angioedema, and then other conditions need to be considered. These include vasovagal syncopal reactions, myocardial infarction, arrhythmia, pulmonary embolism and epileptic seizure. The development of acute urticaria, angioedema or respiratory arrest in severe asthma makes it difficult to distinguish from anaphylaxis.

Anaphylactoid reactions to radiographic contrast media and to aspirin present with similar clinical pictures. They are not associated with IgE mechanisms and therefore cannot be diagnosed or predicted by skin prick testing.

Causes of anaphylaxis

Virtually any substance can cause anaphylaxis but some are particularly likely to be involved. The offending agent can be introduced by any route including inhalation and contact, although the most severe reactions tend to follow parenteral introduction of the allergen as occurs in drug reactions and insect stings.

Drugs are among the most common causes of anaphylaxis, with antibiotics being the chief offenders. Penicillin is still claimed to be the most frequent cause of anaphylaxis. Injection is the most likely route of administration of a drug to cause a reaction. Heterologous antisera are rarely used in modern practice but should be preceded by skin testing. Their main indications are for the treatment of snake and spider bites, and rejection of organ transplants.

Foods are also a common cause of anaphylaxis. Most foods have been incriminated at some time, but the most common offenders are listed in the

TABLE 16.1 **Causes of anaphylaxis**

Drugs
   Antimicrobial agents—penicillins, cotrimoxazole and other sulphonamides,
     cephalosporins, vancomycin, tetracyclines, nitrofurantoin, pentamidine
   Aspirin, non-steroidal anti-inflammatory agents, narcotics
   Anaesthetic agents—thiopental, succinylcholine, d-tubocurarine
Foods
   Peanuts
   Shellfish
   Nuts
   Sunflower seeds
   Legumes—peas, beans
   Berries
   Milk
   Eggs
Insect stings
   Hymenoptera (especially bees and wasps)
   Jack jumper ant
Enzymes
   Chymopapain
   Streptokinase
Biological products
   Blood and blood products
   Allergen extracts
   Hormones—insulin, methylprednisolone, ACTH, synthetic ACTH
   Vaccines, antitoxins
Miscellaneous agents
   Radiographic contrast media (anaphylactoid)
   Dextran
Contactants
   Latex
   Insect repellants (DEET, diethyl-meta-toluamide)
   Bacitracin ointment
   Semen
Exercise induced anaphylaxis
Recurrent idiopathic anaphylaxis syndrome.

table. Foods can induce anaphylaxis by ingestion, contact as occurs in food
preparation, and even inhalation. Skin testing with food extracts is a useful
confirmatory diagnostic test but care must be taken as it can induce a
generalised reaction. Cooking and processing can render a food non-
allergenic. Sometimes exercise induces anaphylaxis after ingestion of certain
foods although they can be tolerated without exercise, and exercise on its own
may not produce a reaction.

Most anaphylactic reactions to *blood products* are unexplained. Rarely
can a food or drug in the donor plasma induce a reaction in a susceptible
recipient, or can a recipient be passively sensitised by transfused IgE. Anti-
IgA antibodies are present in about 40% of subjects with selective IgA deficiency and can induce a reaction to traces of IgA in transfused blood or in
blood products such as gamma-globulin preparations.

Plasma expanders composed of gelatins or dextrans can induce serious reactions, either through anaphylaxis or anaphylactoid reactions. Protamine sulphate, used to reverse heparin anticoagulation, can induce anaphylaxis, with diabetic patients who receive protamine-containing insulin preparations being at particular risk.

Anaphylaxis occurs in relation to *general anaesthetics* in 1 in 5,000 to 15,000 operations, with deaths reported from 0.05 to 6%. Muscle relaxants such as alcuronium are the chief offenders, although it is becoming recognised that allergy to latex in some patients is responsible, especially those at high risk such as children with spina bifida where repeated catheterisations have been required.

In idiopathic anaphylaxis there is no obvious precipitant. Many of these patients are atopic but a specific allergen cannot be identified. Anaphylaxis can occur during or shortly after *exercise*. In a proportion of these patients it is related to ingestion of certain foods which can be tolerated without exercise.

Acute management

The acute phase of anaphylaxis is a medical emergency. In extreme cases death can occur within minutes. The syndrome becomes more refractory to treatment the longer the delay in initiating treatment and the prognosis is directly related to the delay in reversing the syndrome. A brief history can be obtained from the patient and companions but it must not delay the start of resuscitation measures.

Adrenaline is indicated as the specific treatment to reverse the syndrome. It is rapidly absorbed from subcutaneous sites and onset of action is

TABLE 16.2 **Acute management of anaphylaxis**

Establish an airway	
Give adrenaline 1 : 1,000	0.5 ml subcutaneously, OR 0.3 ml at site of injection/sting and 0.3 ml remotely, OR 10 puffs Medi-Haler Epi Repeat after 10 minutes if necessary
OR	
Give adrenaline 1 : 10,000	1 ml in 100 ml saline IV over 20 minutes with failure of circulation or if patient collapsed
Give oxygen	
Establish IV line	
	Intravenous fluids. 1 litre N saline followed by colloid solutions, e.g. Haemaccel to maintain blood pressure
	Hydrocortisone 200 mg IV 6-hourly for 24 hours, followed by reducing doses of oral prednisone if appropriate
	Promethazine or diphenhydramine 25 mg IV
Give oral antihistamines, e.g. terfenadine 60 mg or promethazine 25 mg.	

comparable with intramuscular injection. The dose in adults is 0.5 ml of 1:1,000, repeated in 5 to 10 minutes if necessary. If an insect sting or injection of a drug is the initiating event, 0.3 ml can be given at the site of the sting or injection with the remainder at a different site. This slows down absorption by producing vasoconstriction. A paediatric dose is 0.2 to 0.3 ml.

Adrenaline should be given intravenously if there is circulatory collapse. The dose is 1 ml of 1:10,000 in 100 ml saline IV over 20 minutes. Note the dilution. It is highly dangerous to give the subcutaneous/intramuscular preparation undiluted intravenously and extra care should be taken with intravenous infusions to ensure that the correct dilution is used.

The two features of anaphylaxis which threaten life most directly are respiratory obstruction and circulatory collapse. Attention must be paid to these aspects at the same time as giving adrenaline. With respiratory obstruction it is necessary to establish an airway quickly. Angioedema tends to subside rapidly after administration of adrenaline. It is vital to get an intravenous line in situ as quickly as possible, even if the patient does not appear to need one at the time. The problem is that circulatory collapse can develop rapidly and then it becomes technically difficult to get venous access. An intravenous line is vital for administration of fluids and drugs.

With signs of circulatory collapse such as tachycardia and hypotension, give intravenous fluids. Initially normal saline will do but change to colloidal solutions as soon as they are available. The first litre should be given over 15 minutes, and thereafter as dictated by circumstances. Usually 3 to 4 litres are required in the first 6 hours.

Corticosteroids are valuable for stabilising the situation and preventing a second 'wave' of collapse which sometimes occurs several hours later. Hydrocortisone 200 mg IV is given through the intravenous line and is repeated 6 hourly for 24 hours, at which time a decision is made on continuing intravenous therapy or changing to oral prednisone in equivalent dosages. Corticosteroids should be withdrawn rapidly over a few days once the syndrome has subsided.

Antihistamines are useful especially where there is urticaria which can cause considerable discomfort from intense itching. Parenteral preparations are best under these circumstances, for example 25 to 50 mg of promethazine or diphenhydramine.

Close medical observation is required for at least 24 hours since the syndrome may recur and require further active intervention. It is unwise to send a patient home from hospital in under 24 hours.

Interval management

Once the patient's condition is stabilised, the underlying cause and risk factors for development of anaphylaxis must be identified and addressed. Preventive measures should be instituted to avoid futher events. These include:

(a) education in avoiding insect stings;
(b) advice on discarding medications no longer required;

(c) maintaining tetanus toxoid immunisations in subjects allergic to heterologous sera, thereby avoiding the need to administer heterologous tetanus antisera;
(d) pretreatment with corticosteroids and antihistamines where radio-contrast material is to be used—this is controversial.

TABLE 16.3 **Interval management of anaphylaxis**

* Establish the cause
* Advise on preventive measures
* Provide warning bracelet or necklace (Medic-Alert)
* Provide first aid kit, including adrenaline by self-administration kit
* Educate in first aid.

Beta-blockers must not be administered to patients who have recovered from anaphylaxis as they interfere significantly with the ability of reversing the syndrome. Calcium channel blockers and ACE inhibitor drugs should also be avoided.

The patient and responsible relative must be educated in the condition and its treatment. A first aid kit containing adrenaline is provided and the patient must be taught how to use it. Adrenaline auto-injectors (Epi-Pen) are the most convenient for this purpose. Preloaded adrenaline syringes are also available (Min-I-Jet) but they suffer from the disadvantage of having large, daunting needles. Adrenaline by inhalation is an alternative route of administration. Medi-Haler Epi is a metered dose aerosol. Ten activations are required for a single dose and this may be repeated in 10 minutes. Deep inhalations are not required as the drug is absorbed from the oral and pharyngeal mucosa. The first aid kit should also contain antihistamine tablets and a tourniquet which can be applied proximal to an insect sting to slow absorption.

The patient must be provided with a Medic-Alert bracelet or necklace with details of the condition, emergency treatment, and contact for medical assistance and details.

When to refer your patient

There is certainly no time to refer the patient in the immediate treatment phase so familiarity with the management of this condition is essential. Once resuscitation has been started and the condition is stabilised, close observation must be continued for at least 24 hours. Thereafter, follow-up is required to determine the cause of the reaction, to institute preventative steps and to educate the patient in first aid management. Subsequent referral to a specialist may be indicated for the following reasons:

(a) To establish the cause of the reaction if it is not immediately apparent.
(b) To confirm that a particular substance is responsible for precipitating the syndrome. This is an essential step if desensitisation is contemplated.

Skin prick testing with the suspected substance is a reliable method of diagnosis, but it can be hazardous in a situation where anaphylaxis has occurred. It is therefore best undertaken by practitioners with special knowledge and interest in the subject.

(c) To determine whether desensitisation to prevent future reactions is feasible and indicated.

(d) For advice regarding avoidance of future episodes and first-aid measures to be taken if the need arises.

Background

Anaphylaxis is due to the catastrophic release of mast cell mediators in many sites. Classical anaphylaxis involves the interaction of allergen with specific IgE on mast cells and basophils. This triggers the release of mediators with the resultant clinical effects. The lethality of anaphylaxis results from its effects on cardiovascular and respiratory systems. Amplification and spreading of the reaction from the site of initial exposure to allergen must involve the nervous system. Mediator discharge from mast cells may also occur through mechanisms other than IgE. Complement activation results in the release of small fragments (anaphylatoxins) which trigger mast cells to release mediators. Because the clinical picture may be identical the name anaphylactoid is applied. Skin prick tests for these agents are negative.

There are increased levels of mediators in tissue fluids including serum and urine histamine. Histamine is difficult to measure for a number of reasons, including the fact that it is so labile and elevated levels are transient. Serum tryptase is also raised in acute anaphylaxis and is more readily measured, so that it is a useful diagnostic test for anaphylaxis in retrospect.

Pathology. There may be few or no specific findings at autopsy in a patient dying of anaphylaxis. Findings include acute hyperinflation of the lungs, pulmonary oedema and intra-alveolar haemorrhage, laryngeal oedema, oedema and congestion of the gastrointestinal tract, angioedema and urticaria. Microscopy shows oedema, sometimes with increased numbers of eosinophils. Myocardial infarction is a common finding in patients dying with anaphylaxis.

Further reading

Australian Prescriber Wall Chart. Medical management of anaphylactoid and anaphylactic reactions. Prepared by Executive Editorial Board after review of information from several medical colleges. Insert, *Australian Prescriber* 1989; 12: No 2.

Fisher MM. Anaphylaxis. *Med J Aust* 1984. Special supplement S8–S10.

Position statement of American Academy of Allergy and Immunology. The use of epinephrine in the treatment of anaphylaxis. *J Allergy Clin Immunol* 1994; 94: 666–8.

Van Nunen S. Anaphylaxis—the allergic emergency. *Modern Medicine* 1995; 38: 30–8.

Chapter 17

Adverse reactions to foods

Introduction

Food allergy is a grossly overworked term. It has been incriminated as the cause of many different symptoms, often with little evidence. Inappropriate and sometimes bizarre dietary restrictions have been applied in some instances, and have resulted in serious problems of malnutrition with children being particularly at risk. It is not surprising that scepticism has arisen about this area of medical practice.

Definitions

Adverse reactions to food include any untoward effects from ingestion of foods which may arise by whatever mechanism. They include food intolerance and food allergy.

Food intolerance is a reproducible adverse reaction to a specific component of food which is not psychologically mediated. The reaction occurs even when the particular component is not recognised by the subject.

Food allergy is mediated by an immunological reaction involving IgE antibodies and is manifest clinically as a typical allergic reaction. Unfortunately this term is sometimes applied indiscriminately to any adverse reaction to food. This confuses the whole area and the term is best reserved for the relatively uncommon situation where a true IgE mediated allergic reaction has occurred. Other immunological mechanisms can rarely be involved in reactions to foods.

Food sensitivity is a term which in North American convention includes both food intolerance and food hypersensitivity (an immunological reaction to food which includes IgE mediated allergy). British usage tends to restrict the term 'sensitivity' to food intolerance.

Food aversion is a distaste for food which occurs when the food is recognised, and which usually results in avoidance of that particular food. It does not occur when the food is disguised and can be precipitated by falsely suggesting that the food has been administered. The adverse reaction is caused by an emotional response to the food and not by the food itself.

145

Classification

Adverse reactions to foods can be classified in a number of different ways, for example in terms of the underlying mechanisms involved as represented in Table 17.1; in relation to the timing of the reaction following exposure to the food; or on the basis of whether the manifestations occur in the gastrointestinal system or in extra-intestinal sites.

Toxins responsible for adverse reactions to foods may be inherent constituents of the food or introduced by contamination. Micro-organisms can

TABLE 17.1 **Classification of adverse reactions to foods**

Toxic reactions
  Contamination with toxins or micro-organisms, e.g.
    Salmonella enteritidis in poultry and eggs
    Listeria in unpasteurised cheeses and undercooked meats
    Clostridium botulinum (botulism) in meat, fish, conserves
    Ciguatera toxin in reef fish
    Scombroid toxin (usually histamine) in badly stored mackerel, tuna and related fish
    Brevetoxins (neurotoxic shellfish poisoning) in oysters, scallops, mussels
    Poisons, e.g. arsenic, insecticides
  Inherent toxins in foods, e.g.
    Aflatoxin
    Inedible mushrooms
    Tetrodotoxin in puffer fish
  Drug effects on reactions to food components, e.g.
    Potentiation of tyramine effects by monoamine oxidase inhibitors
    Disulfiram interaction with alcohol to produce flushing and nausea.
Intolerance
  Pharmacological reactions to:
    Additives, e.g. dyes, benzoates, tartrazine, salicylates, monosodium glutamate (MSG)
    Natural constituents, e.g. caffeine, vasoactive amines such as:
      tyramine, histamine, serotonin, phenylethylamine, tryptamine, lectins
  Inborn errors of metabolism
    Favism due to G-6-PD deficiency
  Enzyme deficiencies
    Primary, e.g. lactase, fructase
    Induced, e.g. lactase, following gastroenteritis, giardiasis, surgery
      11β-hydroxysteroid dehydrogenase by liquorice, resulting in inhibition of the renin-aldosterone system with sodium and water retention, hypertension, and hypokalaemia.
  Irritants, e.g. curry.
Immunological reactions
  Allergy
  Hypersensitivity
  Gluten intolerance, with coeliac disease
  Immune complexes following absorption of food proteins. Clinical significance unclear
Psychological reactions
  Aversion
  Eating disorders.

lead to disease either by infection, for example salmonellosis or listeriosis, or by production of toxins in the food, for example botulism.

Food intolerance is caused by additives such as dyes, artificial flavourings and preservatives which induce pharmacological reactions in some patients. Some of these chemicals are in fact natural constituents of some foods such as salicylates in various fruits. In some cases an inborn error of metabolism can be demonstrated such as favism due to glucose-6-phosphate dehydrogenase deficiency, but more often the mechanism of the reaction is obscure. The onset of food intolerance is often delayed for anything from several to 24 hours after ingestion, which makes it very difficult to make a connection between a particular food and the onset of symptoms. Furthermore, the reaction is induced by various foods which are seemingly unrelated but which contain common substances. Food additives fulfill a valuable function in modern society by preserving foods and making them attractive, and in the vast majority of people they are harmless. Urticaria and/or angioedema are the most definite presentations of food intolerance but a variety of other symptoms including chronic fatigue, behavioural disturbances, irritable bowel syndrome and migraine have been ascribed to it with varying degrees of credibility.

Immunological reactions to foods are relatively uncommon. The most widely accepted and best studied are those produced by specific IgE, the classical food allergy syndromes. Allergic reactions usually occur within minutes up to a few hours after ingestion, which makes the connection easier to establish. Patients are often atopic, the reaction is usually to a single food, the identity of the food is clear and the clinical manifestations are characteristic of an allergic reaction. Allergic reactions are most likely to occur in children and infants.

Psychological aversions to food may arise through previous unpleasant associations or because of deeper psychological disturbances which can result in abnormal eating patterns such as anorexia nervosa and bulimia.

Clinical manifestations

Adverse reactions to food may occur immediately after ingestion or may be delayed for up to 24 hours. Immediate reactions are usually due to food allergy mediated through specific IgE antibodies, while delayed reactions are more likely to be the result of other mechanisms.

TABLE 17.2 **Time scale of adverse reactions to foods**

Immediate reaction	usually IgE mediated food easily identified usually a single food item patient is often atopic
Delayed reaction	multiple mechanisms involved difficult to diagnose difficult to identify responsible food components often several foods involved may be a single component of different foods.

Presentation of adverse reactions to foods

How adverse reactions to foods present clinically depends on several different factors, including the age of the patient, the nature of the reaction and the food component involved. Manifestations may involve the gastro-intestinal system, may be primarily outside the gastro-intestinal system or both.

In infants. Infants may present with a rash, especially around the mouth, and/or with irritability, crying, diarrhoea, vomiting, failure to gain weight and wheezing. Food allergy may contribute to the onset of atopic eczema, especially in this age group.

In children. The presentation of allergic conditions such as asthma or eczema may be the reason for considering food allergy. Food intolerance is starting to become an issue in this age group. The mother may notice an association of symptoms such as wheezing or a cough, with the ingestion of certain foods, for example lollies, cordials or after birthday parties. Children are sometimes brought to the doctor to determine whether adverse reactions to foods may be responsible for the onset of behavioural disturbances.

In adults. One of the major reasons for considering adverse reactions to foods is the presence of chronic urticaria and/or angioedema. Patients may also suspect that foods are contributing to respiratory allergies such as asthma or rhinitis. While asthma may on occasions be precipitated by foods, the same hardly ever applies to allergic rhinitis. On other occasions they may feel that certain non-specific symptoms follow ingestion of particular foods, and they seek confirmation, or they may wish to know whether other food-stuffs are also involved. Sometimes they will already have been on some form of restrictive diet.

With allergic reactions the onset occurs rapidly after ingestion of the food. Often the first indication is the onset of stinging or burning of the lips or mouth, followed by itching of the throat. Anaphylaxis may follow rapidly. Other extra-intestinal manifestations include urticaria and angioedema, eczema and wheezing. Gastro-intestinal manifestations are diarrhoea, cramps and nausea with vomiting. Although allergic reactions can be associated with any food, a limited number are most commonly involved. These are milk,

TABLE 17.3 **Clinical manifestations of adverse reactions to foods**

Proof of association with food	Strong	Weak or Occasional
Gastro-intestinal	Swelling of lips or mouth	Aphthous ulcers
	Abdominal distension	Eosinophilic gastroenteropathy
	Diarrhoea	Intestinal protein loss
	Vomiting	Steatorrhoea
	Coeliac disease	Irritable bowel syndrome
Extra-intestinal	Angioedema	Eczema
	Urticaria	Migraine
	Anaphylaxis	Rhinitis
	Asthma	

eggs, nuts, peanuts, shellfish and soya. Allergic reactions to milk and eggs are often transient and disappear during childhood, whereas allergies to peanuts and shellfish tend to persist throughout life.

Most allergic reactions occur following ingestion but touching or inhaling the material can also induce allergic reactions. Heat treatment may render the food innocuous by reducing the antigenicity of the food or altering the offending constituent so that it is no longer pharmacologically active. This is seen commonly with fruits, where cooked fruit can be tolerated, but not raw. Less commonly the opposite applies. There may also be alterations in food with storage. This can have the effect of reducing (or increasing) the tendency of the food to induce a reaction. Rockmelon (cantaloupe) when it becomes overripe, has increased alcohol content and has been reported to produce adverse reactions in patients allergic to alcohol.

Symptoms ascribed to food intolerance are often highly variable, and several different foods may be implicated through their content of the same component such as colouring agent, preservative or salicylate.

Some syndromes associated with adverse reactions to foods

Cows' milk allergy

Cows' milk allergy is essentially a disease of infancy. Most children grow out of the condition so that it is uncommon by the age of 5 years and very rare in adult life.

The onset of the syndrome coincides with the introduction of cows' milk to the diet, which in the case of breastfed babies is usually after 3 months of age. Occasionally breastfed infants can react to cows' milk proteins in breast milk derived from the mother's diet. The onset in infants fed on cows' milk formula is usually within the first 3 months of life. Prevalence is probably in the order of 2% of infants, but accurate figures are difficult to obtain because of the difficulties in interpreting symptoms reported by parents without confirmation by cows' milk challenge.

Clinical presentation

Infants develop a rash around the mouth, or more extensive atopic eczema, wheezing or coughing, irritability, vomiting and frequent loose stools, and there may be failure to thrive. Three typical responses to milk challenge have been clearly defined in a study of 100 infants and children with cows' milk allergy by Hill and his colleagues in 1984 (see Further Reading). They are:

1. *Early skin reaction group.* Symptoms start within 45 minutes of challenge with cows' milk. The main feature is a rash around the mouth. Other common reactions are angioedema, urticaria, wheeze or cough, rhinitis and vomiting. Sometimes there is more extensive atopic eczema, pallor, loose stools, irritability or stridor. The skin prick test to cows' milk proteins is almost always positive.

2. *Early gut reaction group.* From 45 minutes to 20 hours after challenge there is vomiting, frequent loose stools, pallor and irritability, and less

commonly other atopic features may develop, including rhinitis, eczema, urticaria and angioedema, and bronchospasm. About one third of infants in this group have positive skin prick test.

3. *Late reaction group.* These children tend to be older, presenting over the age of 6 months. Most commonly they develop frequent loose stools, but there may be deterioration of eczema or other features similar to the other groups. Positive skin tests to cows' milk are found in about 20% of this group, and these are the children with atopic eczema.

One should suspect cows' milk allergy if:

(a) onset of symptoms coincides with the introduction of cows' milk to the diet;

(b) symptoms follow cows' milk administration. This may not be appreciated initially by the mother;

(c) the child is atopic with other allergic manifestations, especially a persistent perioral rash, atopic eczema, wheezing or cough, urticaria and angioedema, or rhinitis;

(d) there is a family history of cows' milk allergy.

Cows' milk contains at least 25 immunogenic proteins, including casein, α-lactoglobulin, β-lactoglobulin, casein, and bovine serum proteins. There is considerable cross-reactivity between cows', goats' and sheep's milk, but not with human milk, so it is unlikely that an infant allergic to cows' milk would be able to tolerate goats' or sheep's milk. Heat treatment alters the antigenicity of the more heat labile proteins. However, other milk proteins, and especially casein, are resistant to heating. Heat treatment, therefore, is not a reliable method of rendering milk non-allergenic.

Differential diagnosis

Lactose intolerance gives rise to gastrointestinal symptoms similar to those of cows' milk allergy and may co-exist with it, for example after an episode of gastroenteritis. Both conditions improve with exclusion of milk proteins from the diet. Lactose intolerance can be diagnosed by finding reducing substances in the stool with Clinitest tablets.

Other causes of diarrhoea, colic and vomiting in infancy have to be excluded. These include feeding disorders, enteral and parenteral infections, gastro-oesophageal reflux, coeliac disease, cystic fibrosis, intussusception and pyloric stenosis.

Diagnosis

An accurate diagnosis is essential and great harm can be done to patients by placing them on ill-conceived diets for inappropriate reasons. Milk is a major source of calcium in the diet and alternative sources must be provided if milk is to be excluded over a prolonged period. If cows' milk allergy is suspected, the most reliable diagnostic manoeuvre is to exclude milk and milk products from the diet for a period of 1 to 2 weeks. Improvement suggests, but does not prove, the diagnosis of milk allergy, and challenge should be undertaken by reintroducing it, except if this would be hazardous, for example if the original reaction was one of anaphylaxis, stridor or bronchospasm. One must always be prepared for the unexpected occurrence of new symptoms during challenge with milk, the most important of which is anaphylaxis. This can occur even if it has not been present previously. David's modifications of the Goldman criteria for diagnosis of cows' milk allergy require improvement after withdrawal of milk followed by relapse after a single challenge. It may be difficult to attribute a late eczematous reaction to milk challenge, and then it becomes necessary to repeat the procedure.

Skin prick tests and RASTs to cows' milk proteins are likely to be positive in infants with an acute early response to milk challenge, but they are frequently negative in those with gastrointestinal symptoms and delayed reactions. Other tests such as total IgE, the finding of eosinophilia and the presence of precipitating antibody to milk proteins are relatively non-specific.

Management

Withdrawal of cows' milk is necessary for a period. Soya bean milk has been a popular substitute. Unfortunately it is not as innocuous as first thought and severe allergy to soya can develop. Milk from other species has also been recommended, e.g. goats' milk. Whether such a substitution will be successful will depend on the component to which the allergy is directed. Boiling alters the chemical structure of thermolabile proteins and if allergy is directed to them, it will improve the situation. It will be ineffective in the case of thermostable components.

Asthma

Allergic reactions to foods are recognised triggers for bronchospasm and may form part of the syndrome of anaphylaxis. There are almost always other allergic manifestations such as urticaria or gastrointestinal symptoms. However, the possibility of food allergy should be considered also when there are sudden, unexplained and severe exacerbations of asthma.

Food intolerance produced by food additives can also precipitate asthma. Intolerance to sulphites as found in white wine, dried fruit and certain fruit juices has been well documented. The reaction can be reproduced when sulphites are given by mouth in a solution but not when enclosed in a capsule. Initial symptoms are often a burning sensation in the throat. One explanation is that the bronchospasm is due to the inhalation of sulphur dioxide produced when sulphites are in solution.

Aspirin is an important trigger of severe asthma in susceptible subjects, classically patients with steroid-dependent, severe, late onset asthma, and with nasal polyps. This syndrome is known as Samter's triad. Other additives which have been implicated in asthma are the azo dyes tartrazine and ponceau, a non-azo dye erythrosine, and the additives monosodium glutamate and benzoates.

Rhinitis

Rarely is food allergy a causative factor in allergic rhinitis. There is plenty of anecdotal evidence that milk intake in many patients increases viscid secretions and may aggravate post nasal drip, although this has not been confirmed by objective studies and the mechanisms involved are not understood. Certainly symptoms of rhinitis can occur as part of a severe generalised allergic reaction to food.

Gustatory rhinitis consisting of copious watery rhinorrhoea, tears, sweating and flushing of the face can follow ingestion of onions and spicy foods such as peppers and chillis which contain capsaicin. Insufflation of ipratropium bromide before exposure prevents the reaction.

Oral allergy syndrome

Some patients with food allergy report a burning or tingling sensation of lips, mouth or throat and sometimes the formation of mucosal blebs as soon as the food in question is taken into the mouth. This oral allergy syndrome is an important warning that more severe allergic symptoms may follow such as angioedema and even asthma and anaphylaxis, and that subcutaneous adrenaline should be administered immediately. The reaction is due to a true IgE mediated allergic reaction and can be confirmed by skin prick testing with the food in question.

Eosinophilic gastroenteropathy

This is an uncommon disorder characterised by diarrhoea, malabsorption, protein losing enteropathy, peripheral blood eosinophilia and iron deficiency anaemia due to blood loss from the gut. There is intense infiltration of mucosa and gut wall with eosinophils. These patients do not respond to an elimination diet and the relationship of the syndrome to food is not clear. Treatment with steroids may be required.

Aphthous ulcers

Recurrent aphthous ulcers are common in the population and are usually tolerated with only temporary discomfort. Dental problems and stress may be contributory factors. These are termed minor aphthous ulcers. When the ulcers are large and disabling, persist or recur more frequently, the condition is regarded as major aphthous ulceration, and underlying causes need to be considered such as coeliac disease, Crohn's disease, and systemic lupus erythematosus. They also need to be distinguished from other conditions such as oral pemphigus and pemphigoid. There is anecdotal evidence that food intolerance may play a role in some of these patients, although this has not been shown objectively. Nevertheless, many patients are desparate, and an elimination diet may be tried for a short period. It has been said that wheat intolerance, not associated with coeliac disease, is one of the more likely factors to be involved.

Coeliac disease

Hypersensitivity to gluten in wheat and other cereals leads to an inflammatory reaction in small bowel mucosa. The resultant villous atrophy leads to malabsorption, diarrhoea, bloating and anaemia. These patients have an increased risk of lymphoma. The mucosal lesions recover on a gluten-free diet. Serum gliadin and endomysial antibodies are useful diagnostic tests, but the definitive diagnosis is made by small bowel biopsy during the active phase of the disease with return to normality when biopsy is repeated after a period on a gluten-free diet.

Urticaria and angioedema

Acute urticaria in childhood is often due to an allergic reaction to food. The natural history is for this sensitivity to be lost over the passage of time. Chronic urticaria is not commonly due to food allergy. A proportion of cases is due to food intolerance brought about by reactions to preservatives and other food additives. However, this has become far less common over the past two decades. An elimination diet is the way to approach the problem.

Atopic eczema

Allergic reactions to food can exacerbate pre-existing eczema and can lead to acute eczematous reactions in highly atopic children. Withdrawal of responsible foods leads to slow improvement in chronic eczema. Food intolerance also may aggravate eczema especially in adults. Challenges with food additives can lead to exacerbation of symptoms but it is not clear to what extent improvement will occur when they are removed from the diet.

Investigation of potential dietary factors should be undertaken in severe eczema. The number of children who benefit from such an approach is in the order of 10% but it is unlikely that the eczema will subside completely.

Lactose intolerance

Lactase deficiency is the most common enzyme deficiency in childhood where it often follows viral gastroenteritis. It may be difficult to distinguish from cows' milk allergy and will also improve on a milk-free diet. Other conditions leading to lactase deficiency include giardiasis, coeliac disease, gastro-intestinal surgery, protein-calorie malnutrition and immunodeficiency states. It also occurs in adults, and is particularly common in Asian populations.

Other conditions claimed to be due to food intolerance

A wide range of syndromes have been ascribed to adverse reactions to foods, usually with less than rigorous evidence. Several of these are discussed in other parts of the book. They include irritable bowel syndrome, migraine, attention deficit hyperactivity syndrome and behavioural disturbances, rheumatoid arthritis and renal disease. A suggested association of schizophrenia with intolerance to grains, and especially wheat, has been discredited.

Diagnosis

Detailed clinical assessment forms the basis for an accurate diagnosis. The aims are to identify the nature of the symptoms, to determine whether they are organic or psychosomatic, and whether they are likely to be allergic in origin or more consistent with food intolerance. Features of atopy, presentation with classical allergic symptoms of asthma, urticaria or anaphylaxis, and a rapid onset after food ingestion make it more likely to be due to food allergy. The onset of food intolerance is more likely to be delayed. A written record of food intake over several weeks can often provide valuable insight into food habits which may not be appreciated or remembered by the patient when questioned.

Skin prick testing and RASTs demonstrate the presence of IgE antibodies specific for the particular food allergen. These are helpful in confirming an acute allergic reaction to a particular food. They may also be helpful in situations such as severe allergic reactions in childhood where a strongly positive reaction may indicate that a particular food could be implicated in the reaction.

The most reliable tool available for investigation of adverse food reactions is the elimination diet. Some diets exclude only the foods which patients suspect are responsible for their symptoms, and in all but the most obvious acute allergic responses, this approach is likely to fail. Only basic food items should be allowed which clinical experience has indicated are unlikely to be associated with adverse reactions. The elimination diet is maintained strictly for 2 weeks, although some workers advise a period of up to 6 weeks. If the outcome is in doubt after 2 weeks, it is sometimes worthwhile extending the period for another week. Longer periods of restriction lead to problems with compliance and may have other undesirable effects such as nutritional problems in children and habituation to an inadequate nutritional intake, especially in patients with latent eating disorders.

If symptoms persist, it is highly improbable that an adverse reaction to food is responsible for the clinical picture. There are two avenues of approach if symptoms have abated by the end of the period of food restriction. An open challenge can be performed with single items of food added back to the diet one at a time every second day. If a reaction occurs, that food is removed from the diet and once the patient has recovered their baseline condition, they are challenged with further foods. The suspected foodstuff is given again later to determine if the reaction is reproducible. The second approach is to give food additives to the patient disguised in capsules in doses equivalent to those taken in everyday life, with placebo capsules interspersed between the active ones. This is especially useful if food intolerance is suspected.

Patients are directed to take one capsule a day and to keep a diary of their food intake and symptoms. If a reaction occurs, the subsequent capsules are withheld until it subsides. If this occurs with a chemical for which sequential challenges with increasing doses are to be performed, the increased doses are not given. Sometimes patients improve on the elimination diet but are then able to add back items of food until they are eating the same food as before the start of the exercise, without any return of symptoms. It is not clear why this should happen. It may reflect the natural history of food intolerance, or removal of the food in itself may have been therapeutic.

If the original reaction was severe or life-threatening, provocation procedures should only be undertaken by experienced personnel in an appropriate setting with full resuscitation facilities, under close supervision and only after careful consideration of the risks and benefits of the procedure.

The gold-standard of investigation is the double-blind placebo-controlled food challenge (DBPCFC). The foodstuff is disguised in a bland vehicle such as pumpkin soup, or enclosed in a capsule, and the patient and the doctor are unaware of the nature of the challenge. Less than half of all patients who consider their illness to be due to food intolerance will be positive in an open challenge with the suspected food, and only a small minority of those who do respond will show reproducible reactions with DBPCFC.

A number of other tests are available which purport to identify which food components are responsible for adverse reactions. These include Bryan's cytotoxic food testing, pulse testing and Vega testing. They have been shown to be invalid and no reliance should be placed on the results.

Management

Once an offending food component has been identified, it is excluded from the diet for a period of 9 to 12 months, after which a trial challenge with a low dose can be undertaken. At some stage it is likely that the patient will lose his food intolerance and be able to resume a normal diet. This is not the case with allergies to peanuts and seafood which persist for life.

With a history of severe reactions the patient should be given an adrenaline auto-injector and taught how to use it. Unfortunately patients may not always be aware of the contents of foods they are eating, and even traces of the offending allergen are sufficient to provoke a violent reaction. The patient should wear a Medic-Alert bracelet or necklace at all times.

Prognosis

The natural history for adverse reactions to foods is for resolution in most cases. Food allergy to cows' milk and eggs usually is temporary, and by childhood and adult life the incidence of cows' milk allergy has reduced greatly. Allergy to nuts and fish tends to persist for longer, and peanut allergy is usually life-long. Food intolerance to food additives and chemicals tends to abate and most patients are able to tolerate these substances after 12 months. Some vague symptoms persist, even if the suspected food is withdrawn, and it is unlikely that adverse reactions to foods are responsible for these syndromes.

Further reading

Bock SA, Sampson HA, Atkins FM, et al. Double-blind placebo-controlled food challenge (DBPCFC) as an office procedure: a manual. *J Allergy Clin Immunol* 1988; 82: 986–97.

David TJ. Food and food additive intolerance in childhood. Melbourne: Blackwell Scientific Publications 1993.

Hill DJ, Ford RPK, Shelton MJ, Hosking CS. A study of 100 infants and young children with cows' milk allergy. *Clin Rev Allergy* 1984; 2: 125–42.

Lessof MH. Food reactions. London: James and James, 1992.

Novembre E, de Martino M, Vierucci A. Foods and respiratory allergy. *J Allergy Clin Immunol* 1988; 81: 1059–65.

Algorithm: Investigation of possible adverse reactions to foods (ARF).

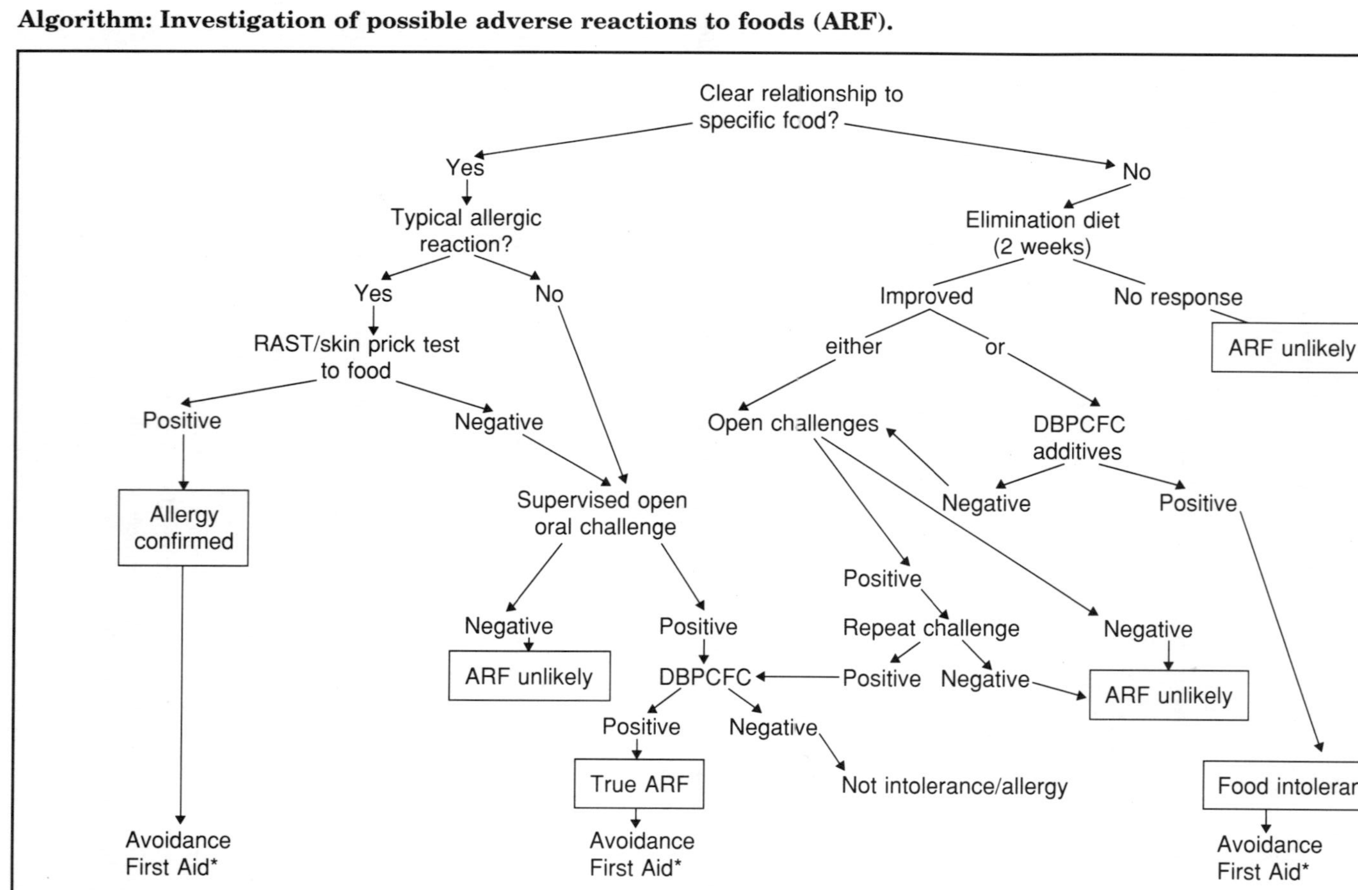

*First Aid: Source of self-administration of adrenaline may be required depending on the reaction. Medic-Alert should also be given.

Chapter 18

Allergic encounters with insects and other creatures

Introduction

Allergic reactions to insects can produce life-threatening reactions within minutes and cause extreme fear and alarm in those who have experienced or witnessed such a reaction. Although the number of deaths is small, there are still more deaths each year from bee sting than from shark attacks in Australia. The prevalence of allergic reactions to stinging insects is of the order of 1 to 3% of the population in the United States and in Europe, and is likely to be of a similar order in Australia. Members of the Hymenoptera class, to which bees, wasps, hornets and ants belong, are responsible for the majority of allergic reactions to insects. Honey bees cause most allergic reactions in Australia, unlike in North America where yellow-jackets (wasps) are the most troublesome.

Epidemiology

Some knowledge of the behaviour of insects enables one to give advice to allergic patients about how best to avoid them. Bees have hives, forage widely and are attracted to brightly coloured and highly scented plants. The imported honey bee, rather than the Australian native bee, causes most stings and is responsible for allergic reactions. Contrary to popular belief most stings occur in suburbia rather than in rural areas. Boys are affected more often than girls, probably because they tend to be outdoors more with greater opportunity for exposure. The most common sites of bee stings are the feet and lower legs. This is most likely to occur when children run barefoot in backyards, since bees are found particularly in clover patches.

Polistes or paper wasps, make their nests under eaves of roofs, whereas European wasps have ground nests. European wasps arrived in Australia in Melbourne via New Zealand. These aggressive creatures are now spreading rapidly up the east coast, and sightings in Sydney and north of the city are commonplace, with reports of stings from all these areas. Wasps gather around garbage and especially empty soft-drink cans. They frequently sting on the lips or face.

Another creature unique to Australia is the jack jumper ant, an aggres-

TABLE 18.1 Classification of Hymenoptera

sive ant which jumps or hops at its prey. It originated in Tasmania, but is spreading along the eastern parts of Australia. It is found in damp wooded areas.

Clinical features

1. *Normal reaction to venom.* Venom contains a number of enzymes and other potent biological substances which cause intense stinging and pain at the site of injection, with induration and redness. This usually subsides over 4 to 6 hours.
2. *Local infection.* Sometimes the local reaction persists or enlarges, and a red line indicating lymphangitis can be seen coursing proximally towards the draining lymph nodes which become swollen and tender. There may be systemic signs of infection.
3. *Local swelling.* The swelling develops over minutes to hours after the sting and is disproportionate to the sting. It may be itchy and red. This represents a local allergic reaction.
4. *Distant swelling and urticaria.* This is a generalised allergic reaction and occurs within minutes to hours of the sting.
5. *Systemic collapse*—anaphylaxis. This may occur within minutes of the sting. The more rapid the onset, the more severe it is.

Diagnosis

Positive identification of the insect should be obtained, although this is often not possible. Otherwise it may be helpful to get a description of the insect and the conditions under which the event occurred. It is important in all cases to confirm sensitisation by demonstrating the presence of specific IgE antibodies, either by skin testing or by RASTs. Skin testing with the venom is more sensitive and can give an idea of the degree of sensitivity. Some patients are exquisitely sensitive and anaphylactic reactions have been reported with skin testing. It should be performed only by practitioners experienced in these types of investigations and where facilities are available for resuscitation. Purified venom is available as a lyophylised preparation which is made up in diluent and used fresh. An initial skin prick test is performed. If positive, this is an indication of extreme sensitivity. If negative, intradermal tests are

TABLE 18.2 **Major allergens of insect venoms**

Bee venom
Phospholipase A2 (major allergen)
Hyaluronidase
Mellitin
Acid phosphatase
Allergen C
Wasps (Vespula and Polistes)
Antigen 5 (major allergen)
Phospholipase A2/B

performed with increasing concentrations of venom until a wheal and flare response is obtained, or 1 mcg/ml concentration has been attained. Higher concentrations will induce an irritative reaction. The concentration of venom to which the patient reacts gives an indication of the dose at which it is safe to start immunotherapy. RAST is more convenient and safer than skin testing. However, if immunotherapy is contemplated it is important to establish the degree of sensitivity with skin testing.

Natural history of Hymenoptera allergy

The development of an allergic reaction requires prior exposure to the specific insect for immunological sensitisation to occur. However, patients may claim that this was their first experience with the insect. The most likely explanation is that a previous exposure resulted in an insignificant reaction and had been forgotten. It is also theoretically possible that the patient may have become sensitised to a similar antigen with resulting cross-reactivity.

The most feared reaction is anaphylaxis. Unfortunately the risk of this developing is unpredictable. It may occur with what appears to be the first exposure or there may be gradually increasing intensity of reactions. The risk of an anaphylactic reaction is greater with a previously more severe reaction (see Table 18.3). Subsequent stings do not always elicit more severe reactions and there is at least a 50% chance that anaphylaxis will not occur after previous major systemic reactions. Various factors determine the severity of the reaction. These include the amount of venom injected, which is determined to a degree by the effectiveness of removing the sting.

Bee sting anaphylaxis is much more common in children than in adults, suggesting that there is a natural remission as children grow up. On the other hand, most deaths from hymenoptera stings occur after the age of 45 years. It is probable that underlying vascular disease in this age group contributes to the greater risk of death.

Management

Avoidance. Patients should be advised on measures to reduce the risk of encounters with bees and wasps. Bees are most active between the hours of 10 am and 3 pm, when the ambient temperature is around 24°C, and on still days. Patients are well advised to be particularly careful under these conditions. Children should wear shoes, especially where there is clover. Patients should not wear perfumes or aftershave which might attract bees, and should

TABLE 18.3 **Risk of anaphylaxis with subsequent bee stings**

Previous reaction	Risk of future anaphylactic reaction
Normal reaction to venom	<1%
Large local swelling	5%
Distant swelling/urticaria	10 to 20%
Major anaphylaxis	50 to 60%

(Source: Solley G. *Modern Medicine of Australia* 1993; 36: 14–24.)

avoid bright colours, especially blues. While travelling in cars or trucks, the windows should be kept closed. It is curious that bees seem to have an attraction for people who are allergic to them. Insect repellants can be helpful for these people, or they can try taking B group vitamins orally which seem to affect their body odour and render them less attractive to bees.

Wasps are best avoided by ensuring that garbage is properly sealed and that sweet food and drink in the open is disposed of quickly. Patients should stay away from garbage collection areas where there are likely to be empty soft-drink cans.

First aid. The bee sting should always be removed carefully to avoid squeezing the venom sac. This can be done with tweezers or by scraping along the skin with a finger nail or credit card. The venom sac has a muscular wall which is fibrillating but which will contract when squeezed, delivering the venom down the shaft. Ice applied to the lesion is soothing and can slow absorption of the toxin. If there is a large local swelling or generalised urticaria, antihistamines should be given. A large local swelling is sometimes resistant to treatment and swelling can increase for several days. In these circumstances a short course of oral steroids may be necessary, for example prednisone 15 mg 8-hourly for 2 days for an adult.

Adrenaline. Patients who have previously experienced a major systemic reaction such as anaphylaxis or generalised urticaria and angioedema should be given a supply of adrenaline and be taught how to self-administer it. Adrenaline can be administered by injection or by inhalation see Chapter 6 for details).

Resuscitation. In the case of a severe systemic reaction, treatment for anaphylaxis must be instituted as soon as possible (see Chapter 16). The outcome is directly related to the interval between the onset of the reaction and the institution of therapy.

Immunotherapy/desensitisation. Immunotherapy with bee venom has

FIGURE 18.1 **How to remove a bee stinger.**

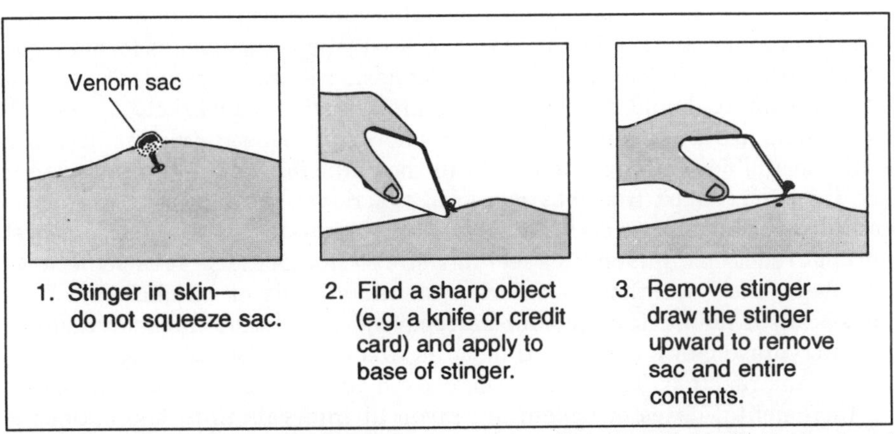

(Reproduced with permission from Solley GO. Insect sting allergy: a guide to effective treatment. *Modern Medicine of Australia* 1993;36:14–24).

proved to be highly effective, with over 97% of recipients being protected from anaphylactic reactions to subsequent stings. It is one of the very few standardised vaccines available for routine clinical use, and this may be one of the reasons why it also has a good safety record. Perhaps a more important reason for this is that it is usually administered under careful supervision and by experienced practitioners.

With bee stings it is difficult to predict what will happen when subjects are stung on future occasions. For this reason the indications for immunotherapy have been difficult to formulate. However, it is generally agreed that an absolute indication is previous anaphylaxis requiring resuscitation. A relative indication is a history of generalised urticaria with angioedema. Factors to be taken into account in deciding on immunotherapy under these circumstances are:

(a) remoteness of the patient from medical attention; for example field workers who may be on their own are at greater risk and should be offered immunotherapy;

(b) opportunity for exposure. A high risk of encounters with bees should be an added incentive for immunotherapy;

(c) age of the patient. Although bee stings are more common in children, the mortality rate is low and as they grow older they tend to become less allergic. Most deaths occur over the age of 45, so there is a tendency to give immunotherapy more readily to the older patient;

(d) fear of future reactions. Some patients have extreme anxiety about the possibility of future severe reactions and this needs to be taken into account in deciding on immunotherapy;

(e) likely compliance with both immunotherapy and resuscitative procedures.

A prerequisite for therapy is that sensitisation has been demonstrated on skin testing with the material to be used for immunotherapy. Skin testing also gives an indication of the degree of sensitivity.

Administration. Unlike respiratory allergens which are depot preparations, the venom preparation available in Australia is in aqueous formulation so that there is no delayed absorption. Furthermore, the material is a purified potent venom. It should, therefore, be administered only by practitioners well versed in its use and in an environment where full resuscitation facilities are readily available. Patients must wait in the clinic for 30 to 60 minutes after each injection. Apart from obvious local reactions, patients may react systemically and require supportive treatment. In addition, they may manifest syncopal reactions, flushing or feelings of extreme anxiety. It is sometimes difficult to know whether these are systemic allergic or psychosomatic responses. If in doubt, they should be regarded as allergic. Measurement of serum tryptase can be helpful if blood is taken about 60 minutes after the onset of the reaction. Tryptase levels are elevated in an allergic reaction.

Incremental doses of venom are given at intervals until the patient is able to tolerate 100 mcg which is equivalent to two bee stings. The optimal dose can be reached more rapidly by giving several injections over a short time period in the so-called Modified Rush, and Rush techniques. The risks of systemic reactions are greater with these forms of therapy. However, the induction phase of therapy is shortened and this is a vulnerable period when patients are at increased risk of a reaction if stung by a bee. The total number of injections is reduced and there is evidence that efficacy is better with these regimens.

At one time it was advised that patients should remain on immunotherapy indefinitely, but it is becoming apparent that a 5 year course of therapy is sufficient to maintain prolonged if not indefinite protection. This is more likely when immunotherapy is given for the less severe reactions and when skin prick tests and RASTs become negative. When this therapy is indicated for the more violent forms of reaction, and where there is no change in skin test reactivity, a decision needs to be taken with the patient as to whether to continue therapy beyond the 5 year period. Effectiveness of therapy can be demonstrated to the patient by having a bee sting him under supervision with an intravenous line established and resuscitation facilities to hand. However, this is an uncontrolled challenge and a violent reaction can ensue which may be difficult to reverse. It should be undertaken only in a hospital setting with full resuscitative facilities and experienced personnel immediately available. Even after successful immunotherapy it is advisable for patients to continue carrying an adrenaline syringe or inhaler with them for use in an emergency.

Stings from wasps and hornets

Skin testing is particularly important with wasp venom prior to undertaking immunotherapy, since about 30% of wasp-allergic patients in Australia show no reaction to the commercial wasp extracts and will therefore not derive any protection from their use (Solley 1990). This is presumably because Australian strains differ antigenically from North American species from which the extracts are derived.

Ant bites

There are several ant species in Australia which cause painful bites, including the bull ant and the jack jumper ant *(Myrmecia pilusola)*. Most cases of anaphylaxis have been reported with the jack jumper ant, a particularly aggressive species which is found only in Australia. By 1986 Clarke had reported from Tasmania 49 cases of generalised reactions to the first sting, with 31 of these developing an equally or more severe reaction to subsequent stings. This ant was originally confined to Tasmania but has since spread into other areas of Australia. Jack jumper ants are black, about 10 to 12 mm long with red or orange legs and nippers. They attack by jumping or hopping at their victim. Their stings are in their tails. They inflict a painful sting, and subjects allergic to the ant can develop anaphylaxis very rapidly. Although the venom has been characterised, insufficient resources have been made available by the authorities for development of a vaccine suitable for immunotherapy.

Ticks

The common bush or scrub tick *(Ixodes holocyclus)* is not particular about its host and will attach itself to any warm-blooded animal to gorge on blood, a process which is required in each of the three stages of its life-cycle. In doing so, toxins present in its saliva are injected into the host. These neurotoxins can lead to the slow onset of paralysis and ataxia. Death can occur, especially in children if the presence of the tick is not recognised. This can be extremely difficult as they have been found in apertures such as inside the ear, nose or vulva. This possibility should always be considered in endemic areas, especially in children with vague unexplained illness and particularly with muscle weakness. The toxin can induce hypersensitivity and anaphylactic reactions have been reported, but they are far less common than paralytic episodes.

Caterpillar dermatitis

The larval stage (caterpillar) of the mistletoe browntail moth *(Euproctis edwardsi)* is considered to be one of the most important causes of caterpillar dermatitis in Australia. The dart-like hairs are highly irritating, leading to rashes, papules, pain and swelling and repeated exposure may result in an allergic reaction. The larvae feed at night and seek shelter under bark, especially that of the stringy bark *(Eucalyptus spp)* and paper bark *(Melaleuca spp)* trees. Children playing on or near the bark can be affected. There are even reports of the hairs settling on clothes left to dry and causing rashes when they are worn.

Reactions to sea creatures

Most reactions to sea creatures are toxic in nature. Examples of poisoning from ingestion are ciguatera poisoning which results from eating reef fish, and scombroid poisoning from histamine in poorly handled mackerel and related species. However, extremely serious and sometimes rapidly fatal results can also occur from contact with some marine life. These include sea wasps (box jellyfish), blue-ringed octopus and stone fish.

Spider and snake bites

The overriding concern is with the toxicity of the venoms, and allergic reactions are not generally recognised. The most lethal of the spiders are the funnel webs (genus *Atrax* and *Hadronyche*), especially in children. Prompt treatment is essential with immediate referral to a hospital where antivenom can be given. Two ampoules are given intravenously initially, followed by further doses as determined by clinical response. The antivenom is a rabbit antibody. Red-back spider *(Lactrodectus mactans hasselti)* can also cause severe general illness with the possibility of death. About a quarter of patients require antivenom, usually for severe local pain or for general symptoms. One ampoule is given intramuscularly. This antivenom is raised in horses. Allergic or anaphylactic reactions can occur with these heterologous antisera. Premedication with subcutaneous adrenaline has been advised by some authors before giving red-back spider antivenene. Other spiders tend to give painful bites with local and regional swelling and inflammation. The white-tailed spider *(Lampona cylindrata)* can cause extensive local necrosis of skin.

Further reading

Clarke PS. The natural history of sensitivity to jack jumper ants (Hymenoptera formidicae; Myrmecia pilusola) in Tasmania. *Med J Aust* 1986; 165: 564–6.

Ford RPK, Dawson KP. Is there a place for bee venom desensitisation in children? *Aust NZ J Med* 1987; 17: 85–91.

Golden DBK. Guidelines for venom immunotherapy. *Annals Allergy* 1988; 61: 159–61.

Hunt KJ, Valentine MD, Sobotka AK, Benton AW, Amodio FJ, Lichtenstein LM. A controlled trial of immunotherapy in insect hypersensitivity. *N Engl J Med* 1978; 299: 157–61.

Solley GO. Allergy to stinging and biting insects in Queensland. *Med J Aust* 1990; 153: 650–4.

Sutherland SK. Treatment of arachnid poisoning in Australia. *Aust Fam Physician* 1990; 19: 47–64.

Algorithm: Approach to management of bee and wasp stings

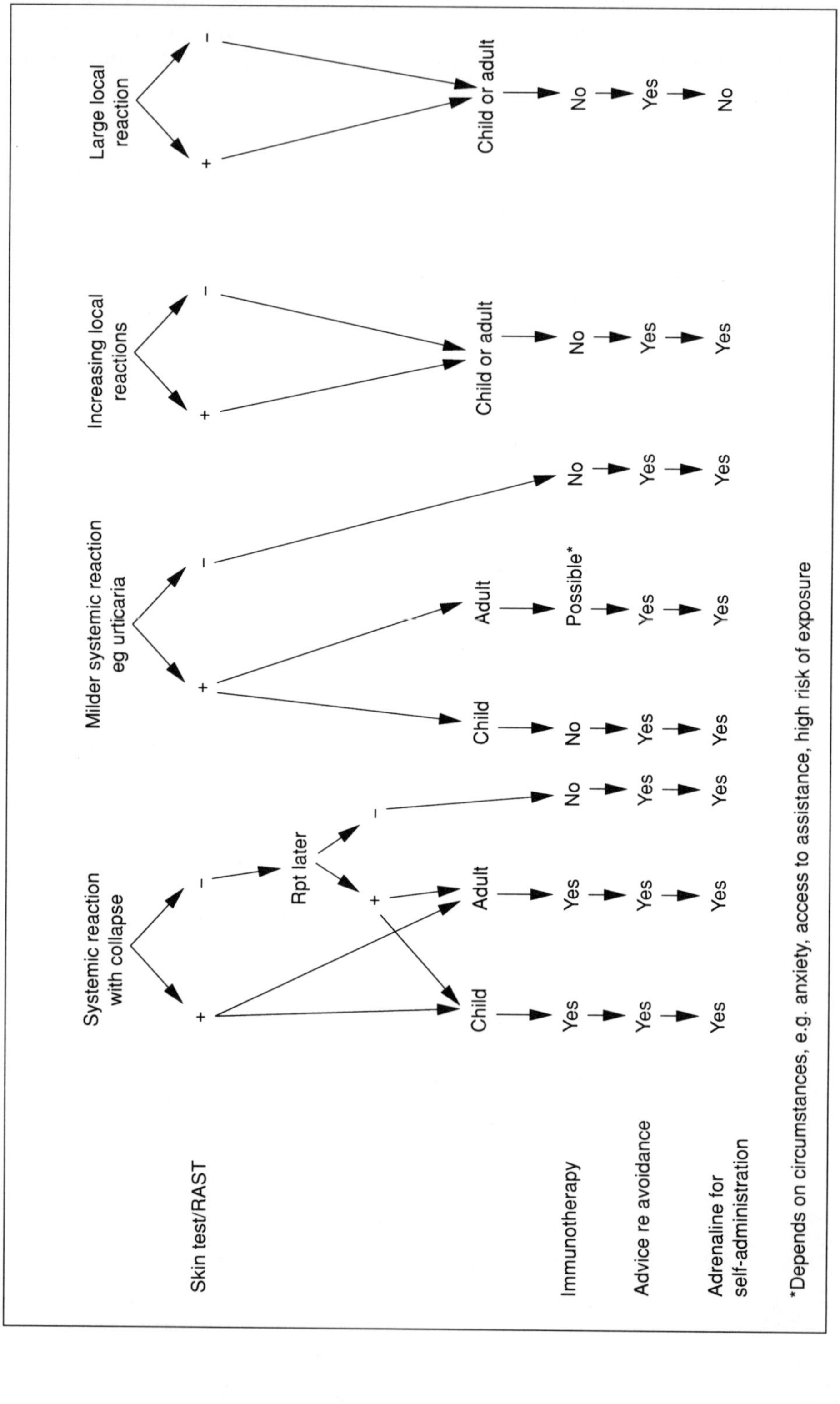

Chapter 19

Drug reactions

Introduction

Allergic mechanisms are responsible for only a small percentage of all adverse reactions to drugs. However, the substances responsible for the allergic reaction are important to identify because the consequences are potentially devastating, including rapid death from anaphylaxis. Often the clinician is presented with the picture of a hypersensitive reaction in a patient who is taking multiple drugs, and then the problem is to identify the offending agent. Adverse reactions to drugs are present in 5% of all patients admitted to hospital, while 15 to 30% of hospitalised patients develop drug reactions which often prolong their hospital stay. The risk of adverse reactions increases with the number of drugs given. It is not uncommon for hospital patients to be on six or more drugs at the same time, and the same probably applies to patients in the community, particularly in the older age group who are more susceptible to side effects. Reactions to drugs can be minimised by constantly reviewing the need for drugs in patients and withdrawing as many as possible.

Classification of adverse drug reactions

Allergic reactions account for less than 10% of all adverse drug events. They are not dose-dependent and are triggered by minute doses of antigen; the clinical picture is similar to other allergic reactions, for example urticaria or asthma; the effects cannot be explained by the pharmacological effects of the drug; and the hypersensitivity reaction can be defined by specific tests in vitro or in vivo to demonstrate the presence of antibodies.

Hypersensitivity reactions to drugs can be mediated by immunological reactions other than IgE. The same drug can give rise to disease by several different immunological mechanisms and these can occur simultaneously.

Most adverse reactions to drugs are due to their pharmacological properties. These can result from overdosage, side effects due to unwanted properties, drug interactions, or failure to metabolise or eliminate the drug leading to its accumulation, as occurs in renal or hepatic failure or altered metabolism in the elderly. Intolerance of the drug may arise from metabolic alterations such as enzyme deficiencies or slow acetylator status. Patients may have idiosyncratic reactions making them more susceptible to the effects of drugs, often for unexplained reasons.

TABLE 19.1 **Classification of adverse drug reactions**

Occurring in normal individuals	*Occurring in susceptible individuals*
Due to known pharmacological properties	Non-immunological
Overdosage	Intolerance
Side effects	Idiosyncracy
Drug interactions	Immunological
Unexpected pharmacological properties	Allergy
Side effects	Other hypersensitivity reaction
	Mimicking immunological reactions
	e.g. anaphylactoid reactions

TABLE 19.2 **Immunological mechanisms involved in drug hypersensitivity (Gell and Coombs classification)***

	Mechanism	Clinical manifestations	Examples
Type I	Specific IgE on mast cells	Urticaria, angioedema, asthma, rhinitis, anaphylaxis	Penicillin Sulphonamides
Type II	IgG cytotoxic	Haemolytic anaemia, neutropenia, thrombocytopenia	Penicillin, α-methyl dopa, penicillamine
Type III	Immune complex	Serum sickness, glomerulonephritis	Penicillin
Type IV	T cell mediated	Contact dermatitis	Topical drugs, nickel

*Coombs RRA, Gell PGH. Classification of allergic reactions for clinical hypersensitivity and disease. *In*; Gell PGH, Coombs RRA, Lachman PJ (eds). Clinical Aspects of Immunology. Oxford: Blackwell Scientific, 1975, 761–81.

It is essential to always record fully the reasons for and details of diagnostic testing, why administration of the drug in question is essential, evidence that full disclosure has been given to the patient and that informed consent has been obtained. Meticulous recording is the best defence in any medico-legal issues which may arise.

Clinical presentation

Adverse reactions to drugs occur as frequently in atopic as in non-atopic subjects.

Rashes are the most common expression of drug reactions. They range in severity from faint erythema to devastating desquamation. There is nothing characteristic about rashes due to drug reactions. They are frequently erythematous, morbilliform or may show erythema multiform, and in their most severe form, Stevens-Johnson syndrome. Some drugs give a fixed drug reaction, e.g. phenolphthalein, while photosensitivity is characteristic of other drugs such as tetracyclenes and phenothiazines.

Urticaria and angioedema are usually due to Type 1 mechanisms. They may form part of the syndrome of anaphylaxis. Angioedema due to ACE inhibitors has become more common with the increased usage of these drugs for hypertension and cardiac failure. The mechanism is thought to be the accumulation of bradykinin caused by inhibition of angiotensin converting enzyme which is required for its metabolism.

Anaphylaxis usually occurs within 30 minutes of oral administration of the drug, or within minutes after injection. The mechanism involved is Type 1 hypersensitivity mediated by specific IgE antibodies to the drug or drug haptens. There is widespread release of mast cell mediators with cardiovascular and respiratory collapse.

Anaphylactoid reactions. The clinical picture is similar to anaphylaxis. However, there is no specific sensitisation and mediator release occurs through non-IgE mechanisms. Examples are reactions to radiographic contrast media, aspirin and non-steroidal anti-inflammatory agents. They cannot be predicted by skin tests.

Systemic symptoms, including serum sickness, fever, vasculitis, arthritis and arthralgia, and lymphadenopathy. Some drugs, for example penicillamine, can induce autoimmune reactions including features of systemic lupus erythematosus, haemolytic anaemia or glomerulonephritis.

There may be involvement of a single organ such as the kidney, with interstitial nephritis, glomerulonephritis and the nephrotic syndrome; the lung, with asthma or pulmonary infiltration with eosinophils; the liver, with cholestatic jaundice and hepatitis; and the central nervous system.

Diagnosis

Drug reactions should always be considered when patients on drugs have unexplained symptoms. It is important to have a high index of suspicion and to document all drugs that the patient is taking. Non-prescription items may also be responsible for symptoms and patients are not always forthcoming about all the drugs they may be taking.

The timing of the reaction in relation to starting treatment with the drug is important. Allergic reactions occur after the first 7 days, and usually from 10 days to 4 weeks. If there has been prior exposure to the drug, the onset of the reaction is usually within 2 days of starting treatment. An allergic reaction is unlikely to develop to drugs which have been taken for longer than a year.

It is also important to ask about previous drug exposure to determine whether the patient has taken any cross-reacting drugs in the past. Cross-reactions may also occur between drugs and other chemical agents to which the patient has been exposed in the course of normal daily activities. An example is the cross-reactivity between quaternary salts which are common components of detergents and reactions to narcotics. The details of previous reactions should be obtained. Patients may report an allergy which on closer questioning turns out to be a side effect or idiosyncratic reaction. On other occasions an 'allergy' turns out to be what their parents reported as happening to them in childhood. Often the details are not available or it may be some non-allergic reaction such as nausea or vomiting. Sometimes the symptoms are due to the illness for which the drug was prescribed.

In vivo testing

Skin tests determine the presence of specific IgE antibodies to the material being tested. They are therefore relevant only for the diagnosis of IgE mediated allergic reactions which include anaphylaxis, urticaria, angioedema and some drug rashes. For the test to be reliable the appropriate antigen must be used. A serious limitation to this form of investigation is the lack of appropriate reagents. The drug may be a hapten and require a carrier to induce a reaction, or the allergenic component may be a digestive product of the drug or one of the large number of metabolic products of the drug rather than the native drug itself. In many cases the antigenic moiety has not been defined, and indeed it may differ between individual patients. There is a place for intradermal testing in drug allergy, in contrast to investigation of respiratory allergy where it is never indicated. Before performing skin tests one must be confident that the procedure will not be dangerous. When there is a history of anaphylaxis the tests should be performed in a hospital setting.

TABLE 19.3 **Skin testing in drug allergy**

Drugs which may be tested for by skin prick testing	Drugs which should not be tested for by skin prick testing
Penicillins	Radiographic contrast media
Toxoids	Aspirin
Insulin	Non-steroidal anti-inflammatory agents
Chymopapain	Codeine and morphine which are direct histamine releasers
Streptokinase	Sulphonamides
Heterologous antisera	Dilantin

Provocative testing (test dosing). Where skin tests are negative or the appropriate reagents are not available and the drug is deemed to be essential, progressive doses can be given with great care to determine whether a reaction will occur. This is applicable to opiates, frusemide and sulphonamides.

The patient must be informed of the potential hazards of in vivo testing procedures, including the possibility of a fatal reaction if applicable, and formal consent must be obtained.

In vitro testing

RASTs determine the presence of IgE with specificity for the relevant allergen. The same caveats in relation to selecting the correct antigenic determinants apply as in skin prick testing. Commercially available RASTs are Penicillin G and V. These are less sensitive than skin testing when the reaction has taken place many years previously. Access to some other RASTs may be possible through special laboratories with research interests in this area. These include sulphonamides, ampicillin and amoxycillin, cephalosporins, muscle relaxants, anaesthetic agents and narcotics.

Total IgE estimations are of little immediate value but they may be helpful in selected cases to determine retrospectively whether a syndrome was due to drug allergy. Serum IgE levels increase following allergic reactions to some drugs such as gold and subside with resolution of the reaction. A significant fall in serum IgE indicates the possibility of an allergic reaction. Other immunological measurements include in vitro lymphocyte proliferation studies as a measure of T cell responses to the drug. Although of scientific interest, these tests are insufficiently sensitive to be useful as diagnostic tools.

In vitro measurement of leukotriene production has been developed commercially as the CAST-Elisa system. It is claimed to be sensitive in diagnosis of drug allergy but its exact role and utility remains to be determined.

Reactions to particular drugs

Penicillin has been the most extensively studied drug. Allergic reactions occur in up to 10% of patients taking the drug. Atopic subjects are at no more risk of developing an allergic reaction than the non-atopic population but if they do have a reaction they are more likely to develop anaphylaxis. Reactions to freshly prepared benzyl penicillin will be positive in only 60–70% of patients who are penicillin-allergic. The penicilloyl derivative is the major antigenic determinant, and when linked to a carrier molecule such as polylysine (penicilloyl polylysine—PPL), its sensitivity is increased to over 90%. When testing with a mixture of minor determinants at the same time, the sensitivity reaches close to 100%. To date, no patients who are negative on skin testing to these determinants have developed a severe allergic reaction when given penicillin subsequently. Conversely, there is a high risk of a reaction when penicillin is administered to a skin test-positive patient. Major anaphylactic reactions are predicted more closely by reactions to the minor determinant mixture (MDM) than to PPL. Unfortunately MDM is not available commercially.

In most situations an adequate substitute for penicillin can be found, thereby avoiding the risk of an allergic reaction. There is a degree of cross-reaction between penicillin and the cephalosporins, least in the case of 3rd generation drugs. Serious drug reactions are unlikely but administration of cephalosporins to penicillin skin test-positive patients should be undertaken with extreme care. Imipenem has extensive cross-reactivity, but aztreonam rarely has. Where penicillin is deemed to be life-saving, a course of desensitisation can be undertaken by a patient with allergy to penicillin. This technique differs from the process of immunotherapy in patients with respiratory or insect allergy which is an immunisation procedure. Desensitisation to penicillin induces a pharmacological blockade of receptors so that the patient can continue to take penicillin as long as the drug is not ceased. Representative schedules are given in Appendix 4. The route of desensitisation depends on the route by which dosing is to be given. The patient must be closely monitored in hospital with immediate access to full resuscitation facilities. An intravenous line must be in place prior to commencing the procedure. Premedication with steroids or antihistamines should not be given as they may mask a mild reaction at low doses and allow a much more serious reaction to develop at a higher dose which is more difficult to treat. Another option is to give the penicillin under steroid cover. In this situation also, the drug must be administered only in hospital with the same precautions.

Ampicillin and amoxycillin. Many of the acute rashes with these drugs are not due to allergic reactions. Rashes are very frequent if they are given to patients with infectious mononucleosis, and they are common also in patients with other viral infections and chronic lymphocytic leukaemia. The rashes are usually maculopapular and unless they are clearly urticarial they are unlikely to be due to allergy.

Sulphonamides. The most commonly used sulphonamide is in combination with trimethoprim (cotrimoxazole) in prophylaxis and treatment of *Pneumocystis carinii* pneumonia in AIDS. Unfortunately patients with HIV infection have a high risk of allergic reactions to drugs in general, and to cotrimoxazole in particular. Test dosing is necessary for diagnostic purposes. If cotrimoxazole is essential, a course of desensitisation can be undertaken but this is an extremely dangerous procedure and is indicated only in life-threatening situations in AIDS. The same precautions should apply with penicillin desensitisation as indicated above. A sample protocol is given in Appendix 4.

Multiple antibiotic sensitivities. A number of patients present with adverse reactions to a number of unrelated antibiotics. It is important to establish the details to ensure that the reactions are not side effects of the drugs. However, there does appear to be an increased risk of allergy to unrelated antibiotics in patients with penicillin allergy, and in one study 21% of such patients reacted also to non-β-lactam antibiotics.

Insulin. Reactions to recombinant human insulins are far less likely than with bovine or porcine insulin. Allergic reactions present with large local swellings which tend to reduce with continued treatment and antihistamines. Systemic allergic reactions are rare and may require desensitisation procedures whereby increasing doses are given until a therapeutic dose is achieved which is then continued without a break. Insulin resistance can result from anti-insulin IgG antibodies. Although rare, this is even less likely with human recombinant insulin preparations.

Aspirin and non-steroidal anti-inflammatory agents (NSAIDs). Severe anaphylactoid reactions with collapse can occur. IgE mechanisms are not involved and skin testing is not appropriate. Most reactions to NSAIDs are the result of a class effect and no purpose is served by substituting one drug for another. Provocation testing should not be undertaken because of the high risk of a severe reaction. Paracetamol is usually a safe substitute analgesic.

Radiographic contrast media (RCM). Reactions are less common with the use of modern preparations and occur in the order of 0.5% of administrations. Fatalities are far less common and a prevalence of 1 in 50,000 has been reported. Reactions are difficult to predict and skin testing is inappropriate since RCMs produce irritative reactions. If sensitivity is suspected, for example with a history of a previous reaction, a provocative dose schedule

TABLE 19.4 **Local anaesthetic drugs**

1. Benzoic acid esters, e.g. 　　Procaine 　　Benzocaine 　　Tetracaine	2. Others (mostly amides), e.g. 　　Lignocaine 　　Mepivicaine 　　Prilocaine

may be required. Most reactions are mild, but severe and even fatal anaphylactoid reactions can occur. The clinical picture is indistinguishable from anaphylaxis, although IgE mechanisms are not involved. One possibility is that it is due to widespread complement activation with release of biologically active split products which cause mediator release from mast cells. There is evidence of widespread mast cell activation with increase in plasma and urine histamine.

Local anaesthetics. Most reactions to local anaesthetics take place in dentistry. Reactions may be due to the drug itself or to one of the exipients or preservatives such as methylparaben. Most are due to anxiety and fright or to inadvertent intravenous injection of preparations containing adrenaline, which produces tachycardia, palpitations, sweating and anxiety. True allergic reactions are unusual but may occur. Skin testing with the two classes of local anaesthetic drugs is indicated. Provocation testing with a small dose is undertaken initially, with increase to a full dose on a subsequent occasion. This is done to avoid the risk of a severe local reaction with necrosis which may develop occasionally over 24 to 48 hours.

Biological therapeutic agents

Chymopapain which is used for injecting intervertebral discs, may produce anaphylaxis in 1% of cases, often after first exposure, suggesting cross-sensitisation with other agents such as meat tenderiser. Negative skin prick and intradermal tests done immediately before the procedure ensure that the risk of anaphylaxis is negligible (Solley 1994).

Streptokinase produces allergic reactions in up to 17% of recipients. Those at risk can be identified by a positive intradermal test to 0.1 ml of 1,000 IU/ml at 15 minutes (Solley 1994).

Vaccines prepared on egg yolk were previously thought to be risky in egg-sensitive patients. However, a recent study from Australia has suggested that measles vaccine is safe in such children and should not be withheld. If in doubt, a preliminary skin prick followed by intradermal test can be done with the vaccine. A different problem is seen with excessively repeated immunisation of patients with tetanus toxoid. This can lead to large painful local reactions due to immune complex deposition.

Heterologous antisera were an important cause of reactions when they were used more commonly, but they are still seen in treatment of spider and snake bites with antivenene and with antithymocyte globulin and murine monoclonal antibodies to tumour antigens.

Further reading

Patterson R, DeSwarte RD, Greenberger PA, Grammar LC, Brown JE, Choy AC. Drug allergy and protocols for management of drug allergies. 2nd ed. Providence: Oceanside Publications, 1995.

Solley GO. Testing for drug allergy. *Australian Prescriber* 1994; 17: 62–5.

Chapter 20

Occupational allergies

Introduction

Since we spend a large proportion of our lives at work it is not surprising that reactions to environmental agents at work are important causes of disease. The major target organs affected are the lungs, skin and nose. Many factors affect the risk, including the working conditions and the type of material involved. Up to 45% of workers with proteolytic enzymes become affected, while less than 5% of workers become affected by western red cedar dust. It has been estimated that about 2% of asthmatics have an occupational component to their disease. Modern regulations have been tightened up and ventilation and protective gear is much more efficient than previously.

Clues to diagnosis

Occupational causes of allergic disease are easily overlooked unless one has a high index of suspicion. The following features in the clinical presentation point to this possibility:

1. An obvious temporal relationship of symptoms to work. Symptoms may be much worse during the week, with improvement at weekends and on holiday. It may not always be as obvious as this, however. The late allergic reaction results in symptoms 4 to 6 hours later so that asthma occurs during the night, and the relationship to work may not be appreciated.

TABLE 20.1 **Syndromes associated with occupational exposure**

Skin
   Contact dermatitis
Lungs
   Asthma
   Hypersensitivity pneumonitis
   Fibrotic lung diseases, e.g. silicosis, asbestosis, berylliosis
   Chronic obstructive airways disease (chronic airways limitation)
Nose
   Allergic rhinitis, e.g. wheat dust allergy
   Anaphylaxis

Furthermore, symptoms may persist in the intervals between exposures because of continuing inflammation.

2. The pattern of skin involvement may suggest contact dermatitis and an occupational history will suggest the possible allergen. Unfortunately, the pattern of dermatitis is not always suggestive of contact. Material can be transferred from the hands to an eye or ear, leading to confusion.

3. Certain occupations are at particular risk of occupational diseases because of exposure to chemicals which are irritant, toxic or act as allergens.

4. Atopy is a risk in occupational diseases where allergic sensitisation occurs. Examples are laboratory animal workers, health care workers (latex allergy), millers and bakers (wheat flour allergy).

Mechanisms of occupational diseases

Disease can be caused through a number of mechanisms, including a direct toxic effect, irritation, through immunological mechanisms, or a combination of these. Allergens may be conventional high molecular weight substances such as animal proteins or wheat flour, or low molecular weight substances such as platinum and nickel, in which case they act as haptens. Grain dust is a complex mixture of a number of organic substances which can lead to sensitisation. These include the allergens derived from the grain proteins themselves, from contaminants such as weevils and storage mites, and endotoxins from bacteria and fungi which can induce fever and respiratory symptoms. These variations add complexity to the presentation and diagnosis of occupational diseases.

Diagnosis and investigation

Once occupational disease is suspected, specialised investigations are often required to make a definitive diagnosis. Skin testing may be dangerous (latex), impossible (with haptens or where a number of derivative substances may be involved) or inappropriate (if IgE mediated mechanisms are not involved), and it may be necessary to resort to challenge situations including bronchial challenge. Part of the diagnostic work-up includes an assessment of the work environment and possibly environmental monitoring. For these reasons investigation is best undertaken in centres which specialise in this practice. Occupational health and safety, workers' compensation and litigation issues may be involved.

Management

Immediate management of the clinical syndromes such as asthma is along conventional lines. Hypersensitivity pneumonitis requires treatment with high dose corticosteroids. The offending material must be identified and total avoidance is essential. The syndrome is not always reversible and long-term consequences may ensue. Agents such as plicatic acid can cause bronchial hyperresponsiveness to other stimuli as well, so that ongoing anti-asthma therapy becomes necessary. Likewise, contact reactions may become permanent despite removal from further exposure to the allergens.

TABLE 20.2 **High risk occupations and potential hazards**

Occupation	Substance(s)
Health care workers	Latex (gloves), antibiotics and other drugs
Laboratory animal workers	Laboratory animals, especially rodents
Veterinarians	Animals, including cats, dogs, horses, rodents
Bakers and millers	Wheat flour
Carpenters	Western red cedar (plicatic acid), other woods, e.g. silky oak (Grevillea)
Pharmaceutical factory workers	Penicillins and other drugs in powder form
Photographic workers	Platinum salts, contact reactions
Plastics workers	Hardeners for epoxy resins, containing phthalic acid anhydride which acts as as a hapten; isocyanates, predominantly toluene diisocyanate (TDI); trimellitic anhydride (TMA),
Farmers	Mouldy hay; dusts from grain, soya bean, cotton, flax, hemp, castor bean, including the use of dry residue as fertiliser; green coffee bean
Spray painters (automobile)	Isocyanates
Variety of occupations	Enzymes in detergents; chemical irritants, e.g. ammonia, acids, formaldehyde; anticholinesterase insecticides

Prevention

Preventative issues are difficult to address. Industrial laws aim to protect workers as far as possible by preventing contact with harmful materials. However, with increasing sophistication of manufacture, new agents are appearing whose potential for disease may not yet have been fully appreciated. Ethical issues also arise. For example, should atopic people be prevented from working in occupations where there is a particular risk of sensitisation? It may be wise, at an individual patient level, to point out the hazards and to advise highly atopic subjects to avoid working with laboratory animals, but proscriptive measures cannot be justified at the present time. Measures to identify atopic subjects prior to employment and to prevent them from working in a particular environment are debatable. One risk of such an approach would be that with identification of disease susceptibility genes such a principle could be extended to risk assessment with other diseases and in other situations such as general employment, with its implications for superannuation and sickness benefits, or life insurance.

Further reading

Chan-Yeung M. A clinician's approach to determine the diagnosis, prognosis and therapy of occupational asthma. *Med Clin North Amer* 1990; 74: 811.

Grammer LC. Occupational immunologic lung disease. *In:* Allergic diseases: diagnosis and management. Patterson R, Grammer LC, Greenberger PA, Zeiss CR (eds). 4th ed. Philadelphia: JB Lippincott Co, 1993: 745–62.

Chapter 21

Latex allergy

Introduction

Latex allergy has become an increasingly important problem from the mid-1980s especially for health care professionals. The risk to children with genitourinary defects who require multiple catheterisations and frequent surgery is even more extreme. The clinical syndrome varies from a contact eczema through the range of allergic diseases to life-threatening anaphylaxis.

It took 90 years from the time that latex gloves were first used in clinical practice, for the first case of latex sensitivity to appear in the medical literature in 1979. Five years later, two cases of anaphylaxis caused by surgical gloves were reported, but since 1988 there has been an explosion in the number of reports, chiefly because of the adoption of Universal Precautions in the mid-1980s which ensured that health care professionals spent most of their working lives in gloves. Gloves themselves vary greatly in the amount of latex available for sensitisation. In an effort to keep up with world demand, some marginal producers released products which had not been subjected to adequate washing and curing, resulting in a much higher content of latex antigen. For some time it was thought that corn starch powder or some of the chemicals used in the manufacturing process were responsible for the reactions to rubber gloves, but there is no longer any doubt that the true culprit is latex.

Latex is the milky sap of the rubber tree *(Hevea brasiliensis)*. Ammonia is added as a preservative, and depending on the amount used, other chemicals may also be added. The rubber is then subjected to vulcanisation, a process of heating in the presence of sulphur which has the effect of improving the elasticity and stability of the product. Latex contains a number of different antigenic protein moieties which vary in molecular weight from 10 kD to 100 kD, the most important allergens being those associated with the 20 kD and 14 kD components. Antigen preparations derived from gloves may contain more antigens than those present in raw latex, due to the production of new antigenic materials (neo-antigens) during the manufacturing process.

Populations at risk of latex allergy

Several well-recognised groups are at considerably increased risk of developing allergy to latex due to their increased exposure to the material. The most outstanding of these are children with spina bifida and with urogenital abnormalities, in whom repeated catheterisations are likely to be required. The prevalence of latex allergy in these patients who have undergone repeated surgery and catheterisation has been reported at up to 65%.

TABLE 21.1 **Prevalence of latex allergy.** Approximate percentages are derived from a number of studies throughout the world

	Prevalence (%)
General population	2.5
Health care workers	15
Dentists	14
Laboratory workers	3
Children with spina bifida	65

Health care workers are also at greatly increased risk. Several studies of the prevalence of latex reactions have reported figures between 10 and 17%, probably depending on the nature of the exposure, the source of the gloves and the degree of exposure. Workers in clinical units and laboratories are at less risk than dentists and operating theatre and emergency room nurses and surgeons. Workers in the rubber industry are another risk group.

There are few studies of the prevalence of this problem in the general population, with most figures being around 2.5%. The presence of atopy increases the risk for development of latex allergy by more than four times. Even minimal contact via skin and airways is sufficient to produce sensitisation in atopic children.

Sources of exposure to latex

Latex is ubiquitous and widely used in medical practice in diagnostic and sterile surgical gloves, in catheter tips, intravenous infusion sets, plasters, vials and syringes, to name a few. There are also opportunities for contact with the material outside of the medical sphere, for example in balloons, toys, kitchen gloves and condoms. Significant amounts of latex are present in urban air samples, derived from motor vehicle tyre particles which get scrubbed off during normal usage. Much of this material is of such a size as to gain access to the lower respiratory tract.

Clinical features

Several clinical syndromes are associated with latex allergy (Table 21.2). A common way for the problem to start is with the development of contact dermatitis. In health care workers this characteristically involves the hands. The lips and face may become involved from blowing up balloons, or after dental procedures where the dentist has worn gloves, and the perineum can be affected following rectal or vaginal examination. Occasionally there can also be local swelling and itching in both males and females when condoms

TABLE 21.2 **Syndromes associated with latex allergy**

Skin involvement
  Contact dermatitis
  Worsening atopic eczema
Systemic allergic disease
  Rhinoconjunctivitis
  Asthma
	Anaphylaxis
	  Intraoperative anaphylaxis
	  Unexplained anaphylaxis
	Food allergy
	  Reactions to multiple fruits

are used. Skin contact can result in more acute and severe local changes with florid eczema, urticaria and angioedema. It can also give rise to severe exacerbations of generalised eczema which is very refractory to treatment. It is important to be aware that skin sensitisation can be the first step in clinical progression to more severe, generalised and even potentially fatal reactions.

More severe systemic reactions generally follow mucosal or respiratory contact with the allergen. Health care workers are at particular risk of inhaling latex antigen adsorbed on to corn starch powder which is easily aerosolised in vicinities where powdered gloves are used. The amount of antigen in air samples correlates with the frequency of glove use and the numbers of changes of gloves. Substituting low latex unpowdered, or vinyl gloves for the affected person, but allowing them to return to the same environment as before, does not solve the problem, and they are likely to develop further systemic reactions to latex particles originating from the powdered latex gloves of other users in the area.

One of the most alarming presentations is the onset of anaphylaxis during medical or surgical procedures. The highest risk is in children with spina bifida who have undergone multiple surgical procedures and catheterisations, with the opportunity of contact with rubber catheters and other instruments.

TABLE 21.3 **Highly suspicious of latex allergy**

High-risk groups:
  Health care workers, especially in theatres, intensive care or emergency and accident units where gloves are worn and changed frequently
  Children with spina bifida
  Patients undergoing repeated operations
  Patients requiring repeated catheterisations
  Industrial workers exposed to latex

High index of suspicion if you see the following:
  Contact dermatitis in a high-risk group
  Itching, rash, swelling or eczema from contact with rubber products, e.g. balloons, toys, gloves
  Unexplained worsening of pre-existing allergic disease
  Recent onset of allergic disease
  Unexplained anaphylaxis
  Anaphylaxis under anaesthesia
  Allergic reactions to several fruits

The possibility of latex allergy should always be considered in high-risk groups but the syndrome can also develop in patients with no apparent risk factors. There are several clues which should alert one to this diagnosis. These include the presence of contact dermatitis on the hands, especially in health care workers, a history of local swelling, rash and itching from contact with any rubber products, for example around the mouth after blowing up balloons, contact with rubber toys and other rubber products, and from wearing rubber gloves such as in gardening and domestic chores. The recent onset of rhinoconjunctivitis, asthma and eczema, or recent deterioration in these allergic diseases should prompt one to consider the possibility of latex allergy. Unexplained episodes of anaphylaxis, especially in patients who have undergone multiple surgical procedures or catheterisations, should be investigated.

A history of allergy to a number of different fruits should also raise the possibility of latex allergy. The most widely recognised are bananas, avocados and chestnuts, but other fruits include kiwi fruit, papaya, figs, passion fruit, nectarines, plums, cherries, melon, tomatoes and celery.

Diagnosis

All patients presenting with allergic problems, regardless of risk group status, should be questioned about a history of latex allergy. Those with a suggestive history, and especially if they are in the high-risk group, should be offered testing for latex allergy. Diagnosis requires the demonstration of specific IgE antibodies to latex allergens. The skin prick test is the gold standard, but there is a risk of inducing anaphylaxis, and this has led some authors to suggest that any skin prick tests with latex extract should be performed in a hospital setting. RASTs avoid this risk to patients, but there is some doubt about its sensitivity in health care workers and other adult populations. Patients with spina bifida, who are allergic to latex, have high levels of specific IgE to latex, and in this setting the sensitivity of RASTs is high. Standardised preparations are not yet available for routine clinical use, but antigens extracted from rubber gloves are relatively simple to obtain and yield a high degree of sensitivity and specificity in skin tests.

In the face of a compelling history but negative RAST or skin prick tests, some authors place a dampened latex glove finger tip on a finger for 15 minutes and if no reaction occurs, a dampened whole glove is worn for 15 minutes. However, anaphylaxis can ensue, and this procedure should never be undertaken outside of a hospital setting and without fully informed consent.

Management

Allergic manifestations need to be treated in their own right along standard lines. However, improvement is unlikely in the face of continuing exposure, and total avoidance is mandatory. Patients should be made aware of the most likely sources of contact, such as blowing up balloons, and wearing rubber gloves. All procedures in latex allergic patients must be done in a latex-free environment. Latex gloves must not be worn by any personnel and no latex accessories such as catheters, adhesives or anaesthetic equipment should be used. Surgery in these patients should be performed first on the list, or in surgical theatres especially set aside for the purpose. This also applies to all spina bifida patients, regardless of history. Affected health care workers pose a difficult problem. Total removal from contact with latex means that they can no longer work in environments where powdered latex gloves are used because of the presence in the atmosphere of powder particles carrying latex antigens.

All patients with latex allergy should obtain a Medic-Alert bracelet or necklace, and should have available and know how to use a self-injecting adrenaline syringe.

What are the solutions to the problem?

A task force of the American Academy of Allergy and Immunology has issued a report recommending that rubber devices be labelled and certified as to natural latex content, that health care facilities be capable of offering procedures in latex-free environments where necessary and that further research be undertaken to reduce the allergenicity of latex products. The universal use of alternative products to latex is impractical at this time. Vinyl gloves are far more expensive than latex and lack their excellent barrier and tactile properties. There are no effective substitutes for latex condoms. Some gloves with less extractable latex are available in Australia, and this aspect should be taken into account in purchasing decisions. Unpowdered gloves are not associated with aerosolised latex particles. The whole question of identifying latex allergic individuals needs to be addressed. Should employees in high-risk industries be screened for latex allergy? Should they be screened for atopic disease since these people have a greater risk of sensitisation than the general population? These occupational health and safety issues are in urgent need of resolution.

Further reading

An up-to-date monograph: Latex allergy. *In:* Fink JN (ed). Immunology and allergy clinics of North America, 1995; 15: 1–175. Sydney: WB Saunders.

Charous BL. The puzzle of latex allergy: some answers, still more questions. Guest editorial. *Annals Allergy* 1994; 73: 277–81.

Report of the American Academy of Allergy Asthma and Immunology. *J Allergy Clin Immunol* 1993; 92: 16–18

Slater JE. Latex allergy. Continuing medical education. *J Allergy Clin Immunol* 1994; 94: 139–49.

Chapter 22

Chronic fatigue syndrome

Introduction

Chronic fatigue syndrome (CFS) has achieved wide publicity in recent years, and these patients often present to clinical immunologists and allergy specialists because of a perception that the primary defect is in the immune system, or that adverse reactions to environmental agents, including foods, contribute to the illness. Chronic fatigue syndrome is the preferred name as it is purely descriptive and has no connotations as to cause or pathology. However, it has been known by a variety of names including myalgic encephalomyelitis (ME), postviral syndrome and Yuppie flu.

CFS is not a new disease. George Beard, an American psychiatrist, described a similar condition in 1869 which was characterised by 'general malaise, debility of all the functions, poor appetite, abiding weakness in the back and spine, fugitive neuralgic pains, hysteria, insomnia, hypochondriases, disinclination for consecutive mental labor, severe and weakening attacks of sick headache and other analogous symptoms . . .' (quoted in White 1989). He ascribed this picture to exhaustion of the nervous system and coined the term 'neurasthenia' which has persisted to this day.

Over the past 60 years, there have been a number of 'epidemics' or clusters of such illnesses which have prompted intensive searches for some infective agent, but to no avail. Some of the better known outbreaks have been Iceland disease in 1950, Royal Free Disease in 1955, an outbreak of the disease in Adelaide in the same year and one in Lake Tahoe in the Nevada/California area of the United States in 1985. The term 'myalgic encephalomyelitis' was coined after the Royal Free outbreak when neurological symptoms were prominent.

Definition

Chronic fatigue syndrome is a constellation of clinical features characterised by:

1. chronic, persisting or relapsing fatigue, exacerbated by minor exercise, causing significant disruption of usual daily activities and present for longer than six months; plus

2. neuropsychiatric dysfunction, including impairment of concentration, with difficulty in completing mental tasks which were easily accomplished

TABLE 22.1 **Causes of chronic fatigue**

Physiological
  Excessive physical or mental activity
  Sleep deprivation
Psychological
  Psychosocial factors, e.g. relationship issues, boredom, lack of satisfaction at
    work, unemployment
  Depression
  Anxiety
  Somatoform disorders
Drug intake
  Prescription drugs, e.g. beta-blockers, first generation antihistamines,
    antihypertensives
  Recreational drugs
Pathological
  Neurological diseases, e.g. neuromuscular transmission, myopathies, myotonias,
    Parkinson's disease, post-head injury, frontal lobe syndrome, multiple sclerosis,
    spinal cord disorders
  Sleep apnoea
  Cardiovascular, e.g. low cardiac output states, postural hypotension
  Anaemia
  Malnutrition
  Endocrine and metabolic disorders
  HIV infection
  Other intercurrent illness including other infections, malignancy, autoimmune
    disease, especially polymyalgia rheumatica in the older person
  Chronic pain
  Allergic disease
  'Fading athletes'
Chronic fatigue syndrome

prior to the onset of the syndrome and with new onset of short-term
memory impairment; plus

3. no alternative diagnosis reached from the history, physical examination
   and appropriate investigations over a six month period (Wakefield 1990).

CFS is a diagnosis of exclusion. Fatigue is a common symptom and can be
caused by a wide variety of conditions (see Table 22.1). It was originally
thought to always follow a viral illness—hence the name postviral syndrome.
However, many cases start without a preceding illness.

Detailed criteria were published in 1988 on behalf of the Center for
Disease Control (CDC) (see Table 22.2) but are felt by some to be too restrictive for clinical usage, although they serve a valuable role in defining groups
for epidemiological and clinical studies.

Aetiology and pathogenesis

CFS is of unknown aetiology. There is no evidence for local muscle disease
despite the prominence of muscle pain and fatigue. It has been suggested that
the symptoms are of central origin, arising because of scrambled messages

TABLE 22.2 **Definition of chronic fatigue syndrome**

For a positive diagnosis, both major and of the minor criteria, at least six symptoms and two signs must be fulfilled.

Major Criteria

1. New onset of persistent or relapsing, debilitating fatigue, severe enough to reduce or impair average daily activity below 50% of premorbid activity for a period of 6 months or more.
2. Exclusion of other causes by thorough evaluation, based on clinical appraisal and appropriate laboratory findings.

Minor Criteria

Symptoms:

1. Mild fever (less than 38.6°C) or chills
2. Sore throat
3. Painful cervical or axillary lymph nodes
4. Unexplained generalised muscle weakness
5. Myalgia or muscle discomfort
6. Generalised fatigue lasting more than 24 hours and following levels of exercise easily tolerated in the premorbid state.
7. Generalised headaches different from those in the premorbid state
8. Migratory arthralgia without swelling or redness
9. Neuropsychological complaints, one or more of the following: photophobia, transient visual scotomata, forgetfulness, irritability, confusion, poor concentration, difficulty thinking, depression
10. Sleep disturbance, including hypersomnia
11. Rapid onset of main symptom complex over hours or days.

Physical signs documented by a physician on at least two occasions at least one month apart:

1. Low grade fever up to 38.6°C
2. Non-exudative pharyngitis
3. Palpable or tender cervical or axillary lymphadenopathy (lymph nodes larger than 2 cm in diameter suggest other causes).

(Center for Disease Control, Holmes et al *Ann Intern Med* 1988;108:387–9)

being received in the brain. Symptomatology is similar to that seen in infectious, and particularly viral diseases, and it has been suggested that it arises from over-exuberant and inappropriate production of cytokines such as interleukin-1 and interferon. This would explain the muscle aches and pains, the sleepiness and tiredness, low-grade fevers and headache.

Clinical presentation

The predominant symptom is of overwhelming fatigue which frequently contrasts dramatically with the premorbid lifestyle of those affected. Victims are often high achievers who have lived in the fast lane. A wide range of symptoms can occur and include those listed in the CDC criteria (see Table 22.2). Among the most common are muscle aches and pains, headaches, tinnitus and disturbance of balance, often described as dizziness. Significant weight loss does not occur in CFS, and when it is present the possibility of other diagnoses, including depression, must be entertained. Indeed, weight gain is more usual because of lack of exercise.

Diagnosis

The diagnosis is arrived at by a process of excluding other causes of fatigue. There are no diagnostic clinical features or laboratory investigations, and heavy reliance must be placed on basic clinical skills of history taking and physical examination. It helps, in seeking other causes for the fatigue, to ask oneself the following questions:

1. *Is there underlying organic disease?*
Interviewing companions and relatives will often give a useful perspective on the illness, for example by providing valuable insight into previous episodes of illness and into premorbid illness behaviour patterns. Features which may alert one to the possibility of underlying disease include:

(a) weight loss—if greater than 10%, it may denote the presence of an underlying disease or depression;

(b) significant documented fevers;

(c) snoring at night and daytime somnolence suggesting sleep apnoea;

(d) specific symptoms such as tarry stools, change in bowel habits or dyspepsia.

Detailed description of symptoms can be enlightening. Headaches of organic origin often get progressively worse, are relieved by analgesics and are not described in over-exuberant terms; true dyspnoea on exertion should be distinguished from hyperventilation; chest pain of musculoskeletal origin must be distinguished from other pathology.

The general appearance of the patient is important, although it must be remembered that patients with CFS and with psychological illnesses may also look pasty and ill, and patients with organic disease may look well. The presence of findings such as anaemia, opaque nails and a rash suggest the presence of an underlying organic disease. Patients with chronic fatigue syndrome may describe enlargement of lymph nodes which are intermittent and transient, sometimes lasting less than a day. However, they usually cannot be palpated at the time of examination. Significant lymphadenopathy is readily palpable and persistent and suggests that another disease may be present. A careful neurological examination is important to exclude the presence of myopathies, multiple sclerosis and other neurological disorders. Urinalysis should always be performed to detect the presence of chronic renal disease.

2. *Is the patient taking drugs (medical or recreational) which might cause fatigue?*
Alcohol and other recreational drugs taken to excess can result in chronic fatigue and a feeling of ennui. Often forgotten is the fact that medications can have the same effect. Examples are β-blockers, some older antihypertensive agents such as methyldopa, antidepressants, tranquillisers and antihista-

mines, especially the first generation drugs which are components of several over-the-counter cold preparations.

3. *Are there psychosocial factors?*
Probing psychosocial aspects can be rewarding. Issues related to loss and other stressors, and the presence of anxiety, mild phobias, especially social phobias, and obsessional patterns of premorbid behaviour, can often give a valuable perspective on the illness. Many patients will deny the presence of psychosocial factors and several visits may be required before they come to light. Patients with chronic fatigue who insist on an organic basis for their illness where none exists, and where psychosocial factors are operating, have a much worse prognosis for recovery that those who concede that psychological distress can manifest in organic illness. Depression and anxiety may be difficult to recognise and are often denied, but the diagnosis may be suggested by sleep disturbances, especially early waking and difficulty in getting to sleep again, lack of motivation (in contrast to chronic fatigue syndrome where patients frequently report being motivated but physically restrained because of symptoms), failure to derive pleasure from their normal social and work activities (anhydonia), and a sense of guilt. A more formal psychiatric assessment may be required to delineate the presence of somatoform disorders and other psychopathology.

4. *Is there advantage to be gained from being ill?*
An affirmative answer to this question augurs poorly for ultimate recovery.

5. *Is the fatigue physiological?*
Some patients make no allowance for advancing age or for the pressures of work and social demands which can become overwhelming and displace healthy lifestyle habits.

Investigation

The sole purpose of laboratory tests is to assist in excluding underlying organic disease which could be the cause of fatigue. There is no diagnostic test for CFS. Immunological changes do occur in CFS but they are not specific for this condition. Deciding on how far to investigate an individual patient is very difficult. There is always the fear of missing some 'silent' disease such as malignancy, especially in the older age group, SLE and thyroid dysfunction. Reliance on a catalogue of investigations to exclude organic disease or to show the presence of past viral infection is expensive and can be misleading. The more tests performed, even in healthy individuals, the greater the statistical chance of finding a result which falls outside the normal range. The demonstration of past EBV or CMV infection on serology is of little significance since these infections are common in the community, and CFS can occur in the absence of a recognisable infection.

Which investigations are required should be dictated by the clinical history and examination. However, in the absence of any helpful leads, an initial full blood count and ESR or C reactive protein, liver function tests and serum creatinine are justifiable.

Prognosis

The patient's attitude is important in determining the outcome of the illness. Patients who are convinced that there is an organic cause for their disability, and who continue to seek it, do worse than others. They often go from doctor to doctor and embark on a multitude of alternative therapies.

Although a minority of patients recover completely to their premorbid functional capacity, most improve to the extent that they are able to resume their careers and other activities of daily living.

Management

There is no specific therapy. The multitude of therapies which have been suggested from time to time attests to the lack of effective treatment. The attitude of the doctor is important. As much information as possible about the condition should be given to the patient to dispel myths like the one that most patients end up in wheelchairs, to be optimistic about prognosis, and to encourage and reward efforts. The patient's co-operation and trust are important in achieving results. Many patients, especially in the early phases of their illness, find it useful to have it pointed out that recovery does not proceed in a straight line, but that there will be 'off days' which, with the passage of time, will become less frequent, and from which recovery will be more speedy.

Measures to improve general health and fitness levels should be encouraged. Depression is common in syndromes of chronic fatigue, either as the primary cause, or secondary to the frustrations caused by limitations imposed by the illness. The newer generation of antidepressants, such as fluoxetine and moclobamide and their derivatives, are undoubtedly far more effective in treating depression and without the side effects of the tricyclic agents. However, many patients indicate that these drugs lift their mood while their physical symptoms remain the same. There is anecdotal evidence that the tricyclic agents may be more effective in this illness. When muscle pains are prominent, patients may derive benefit from non-steroidal anti-inflammatory drugs.

There is no place for antiviral agents, ketoconazole or other antifungal agents to treat so-called candida hypersensitivity syndrome, large doses of

TABLE 22.3 **Management of CFS**

<table>
<tr><td>
• Imbue optimism about the eventual return to a near normal lifestyle.
• Encourage regular, gentle and progressive daily recreational activity.
• Attend to general fitness measures and weight reduction if necessary.
• Reduce workload and other commitments to levels which can be accommodated comfortably.
• Allow a midday sleep if necessary.
• Avoid alcohol.
• Judicious use of antidepressants and non-steroidal anti-inflammatory agents.
</td></tr>
</table>

vitamins or intravenous vitamin C in this condition. Trials of intravenous gammaglobulin in large doses yielded some encouraging results initially, with about half the patients responding. For practical purposes, however, this form of therapy is not an option as chronic fatigue syndrome is not a recognised indication for supply of this scarce resource, and commercial sources have to be used at prohibitive expense to the patient. Because of this, intramuscular gammaglobulin has been tried in doses of 3 ml intramuscularly at intervals of 2 to 4 weeks. There is no evidence that any effect it has is other than due to its placebo properties. Dietary manipulation has been tried on the assumption that the syndrome may be due to food intolerance. While there may be some patients in whom this is a factor, they are a distinct minority and elimination diets are probably worthwhile only if there are other features to suggest food intolerance.

Further reading

Fukuda K, Straus SE, Hickie I et al. The chronic fatigue syndrome: a comprehensive approach to its definition and study. *Ann Intern Med* 1994; 121: 953–9.

Holmes GP, Kaplan JE, Gantz NM et al. Chronic fatigue syndrome: a working definition. *Ann Intern Med* 1988; 108: 387–9.

Manu P, Lane TJ, Matthews DA. The frequency of chronic fatigue syndrome in patients with symptoms of persistent fatigue. *Ann Intern Med* 1988; 109: 554–6.

Straus SE. Defining the chronic fatigue syndrome. Editorial. *Arch Intern Med* 1992; 152: 1569–70.

Wakefield D, Lloyd A, Hickie I. The chronic fatigue syndrome. *Modern Medicine* 1990; 33: 16–22.

White P. Fatigue syndrome: neurasthenia revived. *Br Med J* 1989; 298: 1199–1200.

Wilson A, Hickie I, Lloyd A, Hadzi-Pavlovic D, Boughton C, Dwyer J, Wakefield D. Longitudinal study of outcome of chronic fatigue syndrome. *Br Med J* 1994; 308: 756–9.

Algorithm: An approach to diagnosis

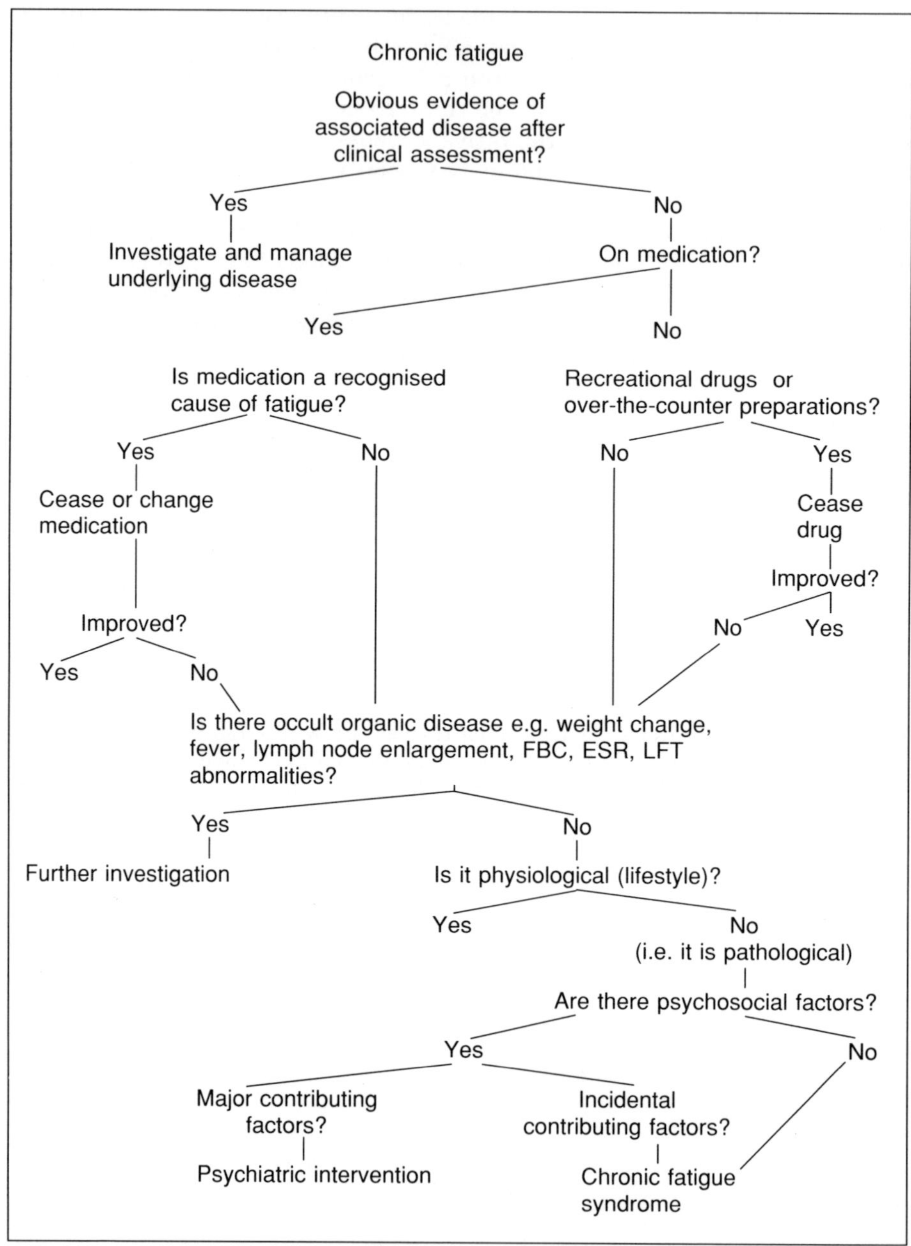

(Source: Walls RS. How to investigate the patient with chronic fatigue. *Modern Medicine* 1995; 38: 115–20.)

Chapter 23

Conditions for which an allergic cause is sometimes sought

Migraine

Introduction

Patients with migraine are sometimes referred for investigation of possible allergic precipitants. About one in three will volunteer that some articles of food are responsible for precipitating attacks. Migraine starts becoming prevalent in the prepubertal age group, increasing in frequency in women during the childbearing years. There is a familial tendency to the disease and atopic subjects are prone to this disorder.

Definition

Migraine is an intermittent, usually unilateral headache, often associated with nausea and vomiting. In classical migraine, episodes are preceded by visual auras, scotomas and/or fortification figures.

Differential diagnosis

Migraine must be differentiated from other causes of headache such as space occupying lesions, vascular disease and musculoskeletal causes. With space occupying lesions the headaches tend to become progressively worse with the passage of time. They also tend to be fixed on one side, whereas in migraine, even if the majority of headaches occur on one side, at least some will occur on the other side. Cluster headaches are a different entity, occur predominantly in males and are due to release of histamine. Temporal arteritis is a disease of older people but important to diagnose as failure to treat promptly and adequately can lead to visual loss.

Precipitating factors

Stress, hormonal factors such as menstruation, and irregular meals alone or in combination, are the most likely precipitating factors. A proportion of patients will incriminate foods, usually chocolate, cheese, dairy products, alcohol, eggs, nuts or fish.

Vasoactive amines can be shown in adequately controlled challenge pro-

TABLE 23.1 **Foods containing vasoactive amines**

Cheese
Yeast extracts—Vegemite, Marmite
Chocolate
Wines
Wattle seeds

cedures to provoke migraine in a proportion of migraine patients. This was first noted when monoamine oxidase inhibitors became therapeutic agents, and they were noted to provoke hypertension and headache when foods rich in tyramine were administered. A proportion of migraine sufferers will respond to tyramine and other vasoactive amines, including betaphenylethylamine (BPEA), histamine, octopamine, synephrine and n-methyltyramine. Some patients report an increased frequency of migraines while they are on antibiotics, probably due to altered metabolism of amines in the gut with increased absorption. The role of histamine is a vexed one. Although it can provoke throbbing headaches in normal people and more so in cluster headaches, given orally it seems innocuous. However, it is formed from histidine in the gut and when this amino-acid is given headaches may be provoked. Although cluster headaches are associated with elevated serum histamine levels, H1 and H2 antagonists are ineffective in prophylaxis of this disorder.

There are reports of some patients showing reactions to food additives such as monosodium glutamate, sodium nitrite and tartrazine.

The evidence that IgE mediated reactions to allergens are important in causing migraine is by no means clear. In some patients migraine coincides with allergic reactions to inhaled allergens and it can be provoked by allergen immunotherapy. However, at most it is relatively rare, especially in adults.

Investigation and management

If there is a strong suspicion that migraine may be related to food intake, a modified diet can be given for a period to determine whether there is any improvement in the frequency of attacks. The strict elimination diet such as used in urticaria is not appropriate as it should only be used for a maximum of two weeks, too short a period to judge improvement with an intermittent condition such as migraine. If migraine accompanies other allergic symptoms or immunotherapy, then treatment of the primary condition may lead to improvement in the migraine. These approaches do not replace the need for other management of migraine. Stressors should be dealt with, patients should be advised about the importance of regular meals and prophylactic therapy may be required. Propranolol is one of the most effective prophylactic drugs. However, being a β-blocker it is contra-indicated in asthmatics and in anyone receiving allergen immunotherapy.

Attention deficit hyperactivity disorder

Introduction

This is a controversial and perplexing area of practice. The term 'attention deficit hyperactivity disorder' (ADHD) embraces what used to be known as the hyperactivity or hyperkinetic disorder during the 1970s and the attention deficit disorder during the 1980s.

Definition and diagnosis

One of the problems is that this diagnosis is often used loosely for any child who demonstrates disruptive behaviour, and this encompasses a normal range through psychiatric disorders to ADHD. If the diagnostic criteria (DSM IV) are strictly applied, the prevalence of the disorder is much less than the disturbing number of patients who seem to be affected currently.

The connection with allergy was started by reports from Finegold that children with these behavioural problems improved significantly when various chemicals and colouring agents were removed from their diet. This work remains controversial to the present day, although a proportion of patients will improve on this diet.

Allergic disease can be directly and indirectly (through the effects of medication) responsible for difficulties with cognitive function and behaviour in children, causing ongoing discomfort and ill-health and by interfering with sleep. Many patients are still receiving sedating antihistamines which can cause drowsiness, difficulty concentrating and irritability. If a patient is seen for suboptimal academic performance, it is important to take a full history to exclude nasal obstruction, asthma and gut symptoms, to determine what medications they are taking, and whether they have disturbed sleep because of mouth breathing or postnasal drip.

Management

Any allergic diseases which have been identified should be treated in their own rights. Sedating antihistamines and oral sympathomimetic decongestant drugs should be avoided. A trial of a modified diet which excludes colouring agents and food additives is often worthwhile for a period of 4 to 6 weeks. This will usually reassure the parents about the role of foods. A strict elimination diet is not appropriate as it should not be continued for more than two weeks. It is important not to lose these patients to follow-up and to ensure that they do not persist with a restricted diet or start a freak diet which may be nutritionally harmful. If there is no improvement over the 4 to 6 week trial period, the parents should be strongly encouraged not to pursue the question of food intolerance any further. Unfortunately there are any number of unqualified people willing to advise on alternative forms of therapy and unusual diets for this condition.

Irritable bowel syndrome

This functional bowel disturbance is common and disabling. Symptoms include abdominal pain and discomfort which may be central or in the lower abdomen, colicky, sharp or dull, and often severe. Bowel habits are altered. There may be constipation or loose motions, or they may alternate. There may also be bloating, flatulence and dyspepsia, and general ill health incuding fatigue and headache. The diagnosis is made after organic conditions have been excluded by appropriate investigations which include endoscopy.

Some patients are convinced that it is caused by 'food allergy', and often particular foods may be identified as offending agents, for example dairy products and high fat-containing foods. Instituting an elimination diet is the best way of investigating the problem. Enthusiasts describe improvement with diets which eliminate preservatives and colouring agents but the data for this remain unconvincing.

Multiple drug allergies

There is a group of patients who present with a history of 'allergic' reactions to a large number of unrelated drugs. Antibiotics are often involved, and patients are understandably concerned about what agents are safe to take when confronted with an infection. Usually the drugs belong to different chemical families with no known immunological cross-reactivity, making it unlikely that the reactions are mediated by IgE. Many of these patients are non-atopic.

A careful history is most important to establish the nature of these reactions. It often transpires that some were not remembered first-hand by the patient, but occurred in childhood and were told to them by their parents. Some turn out to be recognised side effects of drugs, such as nausea, vomiting and diarrhoea.

General advice for these patients is to avoid all drugs, including non-prescription items, unless they are indicated strongly on medical grounds. When administration of a drug is essential, test dosing can be undertaken. A fractional dose is given under medical supervision, with increasing doses at intervals until full dosage is achieved or a reaction occurs. It is impracticable to test for every drug as an elective procedure in order to provide a list of 'safe drugs', although this is often what the patient requests. Where reliable tests are available for some drugs such as penicillin, and depending on the circumstances, it may be appropriate to test for them. Unfortunately there are few drugs in this category.

This syndrome may form part of the multiple chemical sensitivity syndrome which is discussed further in Chapter 24.

Other conditions attributed to allergy without proof

Arthritis

At various times there have been reports of improvement in arthritic symptoms by dietary manipulation, and occasional reports of worsening symptoms in spring with exposure to pollens. Arthralgia can be part of the picture of allergic reactions such as urticaria and in drug reactions, and arthritis occurs in various immunological diseases such as systemic lupus erythematosus and serum sickness due to immune complex deposition. Circulating immune complexes have been reported following meals but food allergy and intolerance have not been shown to be significant factors in rheumatoid arthritis.

Inflammatory bowel disease

Suggestions have been made that food allergy may be important in some cases of ulcerative colitis and in Crohn's disease. Milk-induced colitis can occur in infancy but has not been shown in adults, and most cases of milk intolerance in adults are due to lactase deficiency.

Renal disease

Nephrotic syndrome. A small number of cases has been reported where the nephrotic syndrome has been associated with atopic disease and has gone into remission with treatment such as desensitisation or removal from exposure to the allergen. This is particularly the case with minimal change nephrotic syndrome where a seasonal increase in frequency has been shown to coincide with the pollen season. There is also a higher incidence of atopy in children with this disease than in controls.

Other renal diseases. Interstitial nephritis is characterised by the presence of numerous eosinophils in the inflamed interstitium and in the urine. Many cases are due to drug hypersensitivity. The resemblance of the pathology to Type I hypersensitivity diseases is such that the term 'asthma of the kidney' has been used to describe this condition. There have been isolated case reports of food sensitivity in Henoch-Schonlein purpura.

Further reading

Egger J, Carter CM, Wilson J, Turner MW, Soothill JF. Is migraine food allergy? A double-blind controlled trial of oligoantigenic diet treatment. *Lancet* 1983; 2: 865–9.

Rowe KS. Food intolerance and behaviour in children. *Modern Medicine of Australia* 1995; 38: 38–41.

Chapter 24

Unproven conditions and procedures

Environmental illness

A group of patients present with chronic illnesses involving many systems and associated with multiple symptoms. Some may have recognised diseases, but in most there is no objective evidence of underlying physical abnormalities. Included are some patients with recognisable psychiatric illnesses. A number of different names have been given to this group of conditions. These include the total allergy syndrome, allergy to the 20th century and chemical hypersensitivity syndrome.

These patients ascribe their illness to sensitivity to minute amounts of chemicals in the environment emanating from the fumes of motor vehicles, newsprint, books and magazines, impurities in tapwater, household sprays and emissions from plastics. The most extreme example is the so-called 'allergy to the 20th century' where extraordinary steps are taken to isolate the patient from environmental factors.

A group of professionals, medical and non-medical, believe that patients can react adversely to amounts of chemical substances and toxins in the environment well below the levels which would be responsible for conventional toxicity. It is believed that much of the effect is on neuropsychological function which is not amenable to measurement or objective documentation. The group of patients who are defined as having multiple chemical sensitivities, attribute their illness to chemicals in their work environment. Occupational medicine has not yet come to grips with this concept as they deal with larger exposures and more readily recognisable signs of toxicity. This is a vexed area and has led to practitioners being required to give evidence in litigation.

No scientific evidence has been obtained yet to confirm the existence of these syndromes. The protagonists' argument is that this does not prove that the conditions do not exist and that the scientific tools are not yet available which are capable of the appropriate measurements. There are certainly no grounds for suggesting that allergic mechanisms are involved and atopic subjects are no more prone to suffer from these symptoms than are others.

Suggested treatment has been to remove the sufferer from exposure to the environmental agent. This may include tap water filtration, using cotton gloves when touching print, avoiding foods with preservatives and colouring agents, and even moving from the city to a country environment. It is also suggested that antioxidants be supplemented in the diet, and some people suggest large doses of vitamins. This approach is developed further in environmental units where subjects are confined to sealed enclosures, breathing filtered air and drinking purified water.

It is difficult to give advice when confronted by these cases. Often the patients or their carers have fixed ideas about the cause of the symptoms and the measures necessary for controlling them and it is difficult to persuade them to experiment with other approaches. It is perhaps surprising that, if environmental factors were responsible for symptoms, steps to remove them do not seem to restore these patients to good health. Some of the recommended treatment consists of good commonsense advice and is worthwhile transmitting to these patients. For example, encouragement of regular exercise, a good sleep pattern, measures to deal with stress, a healthy diet and a positive mental outlook. Other recommendations are often expensive with little or no evidence that they are effective, and some have the potential for producing harm, such as megadoses of some vitamins.

Candida hypersensitivity syndrome

A multiplicity of symptoms has been ascribed to this syndrome which is purported to be due to an overgrowth of toxic strains of Candida species in the gut. Symptoms range from chronic fatigue, through chemical intolerance as in the syndromes just discussed, to other features such as feeling spaced out, dizzy, poor memory, muscle aches, constipation, diarrhoea, bloating, impotence, recurrent vaginal candidiasis, to name but a few. The suggested treatments include dietary modification to exclude foods which favour the growth of the yeast, and this includes sugars, foods made with yeast such as bread, alcoholic beverages, malt products, foods containing vinegar, mushrooms, cheeses and left-overs. Other measures include prolonged treatment with antifungal agents such as ketoconazole, immunotherapy with Candida and other mould extracts, sublingual immunotherapy with food extracts, additional vitamins and various other measures. Various laboratory tests are performed such as measurement of precipitating antibody to Candida species and growth of Candida from stool cultures. However, Candida is a normal bowel flora. Antibodies are found in normal people and have no pathological significance.

There is no such condition as candida hypersensitivity syndrome. This is the considered opinion after careful analysis by many reputable bodies including a Commission of Enquiry in Canada in 1985 and various position statements from the Royal College of Physicians, the American College of Physicians and American Academy of Allergy Asthma and Immunology. There is no justification for these forms of treatment, some of which are not without risk such as the prolonged courses of ketoconazole.

Diagnostic procedures

A number of procedures are sometimes adopted which are claimed to be useful in the diagnosis of allergy, and particularly food allergy. The following have been investigated and shown to be of no value:

1. *The cytotoxic test,* also known as Bryan's test, is used for determining the presence of food allergy or intolerance. It is performed by mixing an extract of food with peripheral blood leucocytes on a slide and observing the behaviour of the leucocytes. Any change in morphology is taken to be a positive result. The test is not reproducible and does not correlate with clinical evidence of food intolerance or allergy.

2. *The pulse test* measures the pulse rate after ingestion or injection of the material being tested, and a change in either direction is taken to be positive. There are several variations on the theme such as measurement of skin resistance when a food extract is placed in the circuit between skin and a galvanometer, subjectively measuring muscle strength when a glass vial of food extract is placed on the patient's skin, and other procedures such as the Vega machine and Alcat technique. None of these tests have any validity.

3. *Rinkel's end-point titration.* Increasing concentrations of allergen are injected intradermally until a wheal is induced. This is then used to establish the initial dose of immunotherapy. The procedure is repeated at intervals during the course of treatment. Used as recommended, this procedure results in doses of allergen too low to be effective. The principle of end-point titration is used in determining starting doses of bee venom immunotherapy, but the practice differs from that advocated in the Rinkel technique and it is not used for monitoring therapy.

Treatment methods

1. *Provocation—neutralisation testing.* Variable amounts of extracts, usually foods or chemicals, are administered sublingually or by injection until symptoms are provoked or neutralised as judged subjectively, depending on the particular protocol adopted. The selected dose is then given repeatedly. Given the large number of chemicals involved in chemical sensitivities, and the length of time required to perform one test, the patient could be involved in weeks or months of testing. The rationale of the test is difficult to support on theoretical grounds and there is no evidence for efficacy of this procedure.

2. *Homeopathy, naturopathy and other alternative therapies.* The principle of homeopathy is the administration of minute amounts of the offending material prepared by a process of succussion, which is mixing by violent shaking of a very dilute extract. Naturopaths, often on the basis of iridology, kinesiology or other procedures, diagnose a deficiency of some essential element or an accumulation of some metabolites which leads to poisoning of the system. Herbs and potions are then prescribed to cleanse the system. Because of the difficulty in treating many patients and the undoubted failure of conventional treatment in some cases, many allergic

patients consult alternative practitioners. Anecdotal stories of success abound, but there is a placebo success rate of around 40% in allergic diseases, and one does not so readily hear of the failures or see reported successful placebo-controlled studies.

3. *Desensitisation to foods.* Preparation of food extract injections based on one of these spurious tests, or even on skin test results, is ineffective in allergy and should not be performed. Some patients have been desensitised to peanuts which are ubiquitous and difficult to avoid, and which can cause particularly severe anaphylactic reactions. This is a dangerous procedure and should not be undertaken by anyone without considerable experience in immunotherapy and with full resuscitation facilities and assistance immediately available on site.

4. *Administration of mega-doses of vitamins and minerals* has been used in various situations, but there are no studies documenting efficacy in a scientifically acceptable manner.

5. *Sublingual administration of immunotherapy* is widely practised but controlled trials have so far not been successful in establishing efficacy. On the other hand there have been some severe allergic reactions from sublingual administration of allergen to highly allergic individuals. It cannot be recommended as an alternative to subcutaneous injections.

Remote practice of allergy

This term means the diagnosis of allergy and prescription of treatment based on the results of skin prick tests and in vitro tests of specific IgE antibody without a clinical assessment. Patients are sometimes prescribed immunotherapy with extracts made up of any allergens to which an IgE reaction can be shown. Multiple allergen immunotherapy formulated in this way is ineffective and has contributed to the skepticism surrounding this form of therapy. This form of practice is unacceptable.

Further reading

American Academy of Allergy and Immunology. Position statements. Candida hypersensitivity syndrome. *J Allergy Clin Immunol* 1986; 78: 271; Clinical ecology. *J Allergy Clin Immunol* 1986; 78: 269.

American College of Physicians. Clinical ecology. *Ann Intern Med* 1989; 111: 168–78.

Terr AI. Clinical ecology. Editorial. *J Allergy Clin Immunol* 1987; 79: 423.

Terr AI. Unconventional theories and unproven methods in allergy. *In*: Middleton Jnr E, Reed CE, Ellis EF, et al (eds). Allergy principles and practice. 4th ed. St Louis: Mosby, 1993; 1767–93.

PART C

Basic Mechanisms in Allergic Diseases

Chapter 25

Epidemiology of allergic diseases

Introduction

Allergic diseases are among the most common reasons that patients consult their general practitioners. The perception that there is an increase in prevalence of allergic diseases is supported by studies from around the world which indicate that this increase is genuine and not merely greater recognition of the problem.

Respiratory allergies—asthma and allergic rhinitis

In Australia the prevalence of current asthma (asthma at the time of interview) in subjects between the ages of 8 and 11 years was 4.5% (Woolcock et al, 1995) in 1982, and in 1992, 11.9%. The respective figures of cumulative prevalence ('have you ever had asthma?') of asthma were 9.1% and 37.7%, and for allergic rhinitis, 20.5% and 34%. The prevalence of asthma in other developed countries around the world is of the same order of magnitude, although not as high as in Australia and New Zealand, and it is showing a similar increase. The English speaking countries tend to have higher prevalence rates than other countries. In the USA blacks have a higher prevalence of asthma than whites, and asthma is more common in urban than rural communities. Asthma is a rare disease among developing nations such as those of Africa. This has been ascribed to parasitism which leads to high IgE production which blocks mast cell receptors. This theory has been contested and it is perhaps more likely that the differences are due to lack of exposure to environmental allergens. This interpretation is borne out by experience in Papua New Guinea where asthma was virtually unknown until the arrival of Europeans who introduced blankets and with them house dust mites. Asthma in this country is usually of late onset and there is a close correlation between asthma, IgE levels and house dust mite allergy.

A different issue is highlighted in Tristan da Cunha, a small island in the South Atlantic, where the prevalence of asthma is 22%, and mostly mild. In this highly inbred community asthma has been shown to derive from two or three asthmatics in the original 15 settlers on the island.

The prevalence of allergic rhinitis has also been increasing worldwide as

TABLE 25.1 **Prevalence of respiratory allergies in various populations**

Country	Year	n studied	Age (years)	Prevalence (%) Asthma	Rhinitis	First author
Australia	1992	873	8–11	37.7	34	Peat
New Zealand	1989	435	12–18	34.0	21.3	Shaw
USA	1971–74		6–11	4.8		Gergon
	1976–80	27,275	6–11	7.6		
Wales	1973			6.0		Burr
	1988	965	12	12.0		
France	1982	10,559	21	5.4		Perdrizet
Sweden	1981	57,150	17–20	2.8*		Aberg
Gambia (rural)	1975	231	All	Nil		Godfrey
Tristan da Cunha	1974	286	All	22		Mantle

*Current asthma

illustrated in an epidemiological study from Tasmania. Eight thousand seven-year-olds and their parents were surveyed for allergic rhinitis in 1968. Between 1991 and 1993, 2,000 of the original children were contacted with a 75% response rate. By this time 41.3% of the population surveyed as 7-year-olds in 1968, reported hayfever symptoms, compared with 19.2% of their parents 25 years previously (Hopper et al, 1995).

Questionnaires administered to two consecutive years of medical students in Cape Town in 1974 and 1975 provided some interesting data (Walls, unpublished). Two hundred and fourteen students in their early twenties were surveyed with similar results for the two years. The prevalence of asthma was 4.7%, rhinitis 31.3% and urticaria 8.5%.

Other allergic diseases

The prevalence of atopic eczema in childhood is of the order of 3 to 5%. It is associated with other atopic diseases, and eczema is more common in populations with a high prevalence of asthma. Atopic eczema usually starts in infancy and early childhood and often resolves by the time the child goes to school. It is more common in boys than girls in early life, but females predominate in later childhood and in adulthood. The presence of eczema is a risk factor for the later development of asthma and of allergic rhinitis. Asthma develops at an earlier age in children with eczema. There is evidence that the prevalence of eczema is increasing in parallel with that of respiratory allergic disease. In Japan, for example, the prevalence of eczema increased from 1.94% in 1981 to 2.54% in 1988. It was also found to be more common in urban than in rural communities (Nakagawa & Miyamoto, 1991).

The prevalence of urticaria has remained relatively constant with about 20% of the population having urticaria at some time in their lives.

Reactions to mosquito bites are relatively common. They may produce local discomfort but are not considered to be a risk for anaphylaxis. The prevalence of anaphylaxis to stinging insects is of the order of 0.4% of the general population, with bee stings accounting for the majority of cases. Wasp stings and ant bites are much less common, but potentially very dangerous.

It is difficult to get a meaningful estimate of the prevalence of allergic reactions to drugs. It has been estimated that adverse reactions occur in 15 to 30% of hospitalised patients, but immunological hypersensitivity reactions account for only about 10% of these. Anaphylactic reactions to drugs are the most immediately life-threatening and of these, penicillins and sulphonamides account for the majority. Reactions to penicillin occur in 0.7 to 10% of individuals receiving the drug, but anaphylactic reactions occur in only 0.5%. Atopic individuals are at no greater risk of allergic reactions to drugs than are the rest of the population.

Some suggested explanations for the increase in respiratory allergic disease

Industrial pollution

The startling increase in allergic diseases in developed countries around the world has led to the postulate that industrial pollution is a risk factor for the development of asthma and allergic rhinitis. However, in Australia the prevalence has increased equally in the country as in city areas. Furthermore, with the opening up of Eastern Europe, it has become clear that the prevalence of asthma is much higher in the West than the East, despite the fact that industrial pollution is much higher in the East than the West. Closer scrutiny shows up the point that the nature of pollution is different in the two regions. Whereas, in the East nitric acid and sulphur dioxide emissions (Type I pollutants) from heavy industry are more prevalent and are important in production of chronic bronchitis, in the West there is an increased incidence of photochemical emissions (Type II) which may be more important in producing allergic reactions. A huge research effort is being undertaken around the world to try to understand the role of different types of pollutants in generating allergic and inflammatory diseases. It has been suggested that pollutants may act as adjuvants, enhancing the immune response to antigen in particular directions without themselves being the target of the immune response. Some recent tantalising work suggests that the Type II pollutants may adhere to pollen grains and other allergens thereby inducing a change in the immunological reaction.

In Japan the prevalence of pollenosis has increased markedly since the Second World War. There is evidence that the prevalence of seasonal pollenosis due to Japanese cedar (*Cryptomeria japonica*) is greatest along motorways where there are increased amounts of diesel fuel particles in the atmosphere (Nakagawa & Miyamoto, 1991). It has been shown that this material enhances immune reactions. Another potential contributor to the problem has only recently been recognised in the form of latex particles which are scrubbed off motor vehicle tyres during normal usage. This material can act as an antigen in its own right, or as an adjuvant, increasing the response to other allergens.

TABLE 25.2 **Significance of various types of air pollution**

	Type I Primary pollutants	Type II Primary and secondary pollutants
Components	Sulphur dioxide Total suspended particles (TSP) Dust fall	Oxides of nitric acid (NOx) Volatile organic compounds (VOCs) Carbon monoxide Hydrocarbons Ozone (O3) Small particulate matter (<2.5 micron)
Source	Outdoors Heavy industry	Outdoors and indoors Combustion engines Unflued gas heaters
Predisposes to	Infective inflammation Recurrent bronchitis Viral infections	Allergic sensitisation Asthma, eczema, allergic rhinitis
Prevalence	Eastern Europe	Highly populated industrialised countries, e.g. Western Europe

Other external environmental factors

Planting of heavily pollinating exotic species has increased the opportunity for sensitisation. Introduced grass species such as rye grass are the most common cause of pollinosis in Australia. Other examples are the proliferation of olive trees in the Adelaide Hills which has led to them becoming a major cause of respiratory allergy as is the case in Mediterranean countries. In Alice Springs couch grass has recently been recognised as the cause of peaks of allergy during spring. Parietaria is an introduced Mediterranean weed which is an important cause of respiratory allergy and is spreading widely throughout Sydney. Echium plantagineum (Paterson's Curse) was introduced as a garden plant but spread widely through inland parts of Australia, and although primarily an insect-pollinated plant, it is now known to cause sensitisation and allergic symptoms, and may be important in 'priming' susceptible people to react more severely to grass pollens which appear later in the season.

Indoor environmental quality

There is ample epidemiological evidence for the importance of dust mite allergy as a risk factor for the development of asthma, and this has led to an interest in measures which help to curtail house dust mite numbers. An epidemic of house dust mite allergy occurred in Denmark following the oil crisis of the early 1970s when tight buildings were designed to reduce energy loss to the outside. The realisation that internal environmental quality can have a profound effect on the development of allergic disease has led to greater interest in building codes to ensure adequate ventilation and avoidance of damp, and in the use of the most appropriate fabrics and materials for floor coverings and furnishings. It has also led to the realisation that the nature of some buildings predisposes to an increase in allergen loads and to the release of chemicals such as formaldehyde which result in ill-health of the occupants. This has led to the concept of 'sick building syndromes'.

'Food pollution'

Possibly the missing link in the increase in allergic diseases is the 'pollution' of our foods with the widespread use of preservatives, colouring agents and other additives to enhance the attractiveness and keeping qualities of foods as part of our modern way of life.

Severity of allergic diseases

There is little information as to whether allergic diseases are more severe than previously. Although the prevalence of asthma has been increasing, mortality rates for asthma in Australia for the 5–34 year age group have declined in the 5 years to 1994. This could well be due to improved management practices and effective implementation of the National Asthma Management Plan.

Further reading

Hopper J, Jenkins M, Carlin B, Giles G. Increase in the self-reported prevalence of asthma and hayfever in adults over the last generation: a matched parent-offspring study. *Aust J Public Health* 1995; 19: 120–4.

Nakagawa T, Miyamoto T. Epidemiology of atopic diseases in Japan. *Allergy Clin Immunol News* 1991; 3: 103–6

Proceedings of Workshop Panel. Epidemiological and socio-economic aspects of allergic disease. *Clin Allergy* 1986; Vol 16, Supplement: 11–17.

Samut JM, Marbury MC, Spengler JD. Health effects and sources of indoor air pollution. Part 1. *Am Rev Respir Dis* 1987; 136: 1486–1508.

Woolcock AJ, Peat JK, Trevillion LM. Changing prevalences of allergies worldwide. *In:* Johansson SGO (ed). Progress in Allergy and Clinical Immunology Vol 3: 167–71. Kirkland WA, USA: Hogrefe & Huber, 1995.

Wilson JW, Jenkins CR. Asthma mortality: where is it going? *Med J Aust* 1996; 164: 391–2.

Chapter 26

Biology of the allergic reaction

Immunology

Introduction

Allergic diseases are caused by inflammatory reactions to extrinsic allergens, mediated through immunological mechanisms. The biology of the immune response is far more intricate than presented here, and our understanding of it is increasing at an exponential rate. This is extremely exciting because it is opening up possibilities of new approaches to therapy, some of which may well be in clinical use within a decade. Readers requiring more comprehensive reviews of immunology should consult one of the texts in the bibliography.

Some definitions

Allergy is an altered reaction to antigen as a result of prior experience of it. The subsequent immune response differs qualitatively and quantitatively from the original episode. The terms immediate hypersensitivity, Type I and IgE mediated hypersensitivity, also relate to allergic reactions. Modern usage restricts the term allergy to IgE mediated diseases. The same clinical picture can result from non-immune mechanisms which are described as anaphylactoid reactions.

Atopy defines a proportion of the population who are predisposed to developing allergic diseases because they preferentially produce specific IgE antibody to common environmental allergens such as house dust mite, pollens or animal danders.

Allergens are antigenic substances which stimulate an allergic response.

Hypersensitivity is an increased immune response leading to clinical effects, usually as a result of tissue damage. Various immunological mechanisms are involved and hypersensitivity reactions have been classified into four types by Gell and Coombs. This classification assists our understanding of the mechanisms involved, but it must be remembered that it is artificial, and in 'real life' several mechanisms are invoked by antigen simultaneously.

The immunology of the allergic reaction will be described in the context of a play, with a description of the components as the cast, and the process as the plot.

TABLE 26.1 **Classification of hypersensitivity reactions**

Type	Synonym	Mechanism	Examples
1	Immediate hypersensitivity	IgE	Allergic rhinitis, asthma, urticaria, anaphylaxis
2	Antibody-mediated	IgG, IgM	Haemolytic anaemia Goodpastures syndrome
3	Immune complex disease	Antigen-antibody-complement complex	SLE, serum sickness
4	Delayed hypersensitivity, Cell mediated	T cells and accessory cells	Graft rejection, infections with intra-cellular pathogens, e.g. M tb, M leprae

The cast

Cells

Lymphocytes. These are the 'intelligent' cells of the immune response, recognising foreign antigens and directing and modulating the resulting immune response. Their uniform appearance on the blood film and in tissues hides a diversity of populations with different functions. Lymphocytes derive from bone-marrow precursors along a maturation pathway which can be traced by the appearance at different stages of cell-surface markers. These can be demonstrated by various technologies using monoclonal antibodies raised to surface molecules. Initially many of the same molecules had different names, but now, as a result of international consensus, they have been designated by numbers (CD or Cluster of Differentiation antigens). Further diversity of CD4+ T cell populations has been recognised in recent years, which is pivotal to the understanding of allergic diseases and the role of cytokines.

T cells are recognised by the presence of CD3 surface antigens. There are two main T cell populations, one of which is cytotoxic to target cells and suppresses the immune response. These bear CD8 surface markers. The other population is known as the helper/inducer cell population and carry the CD4 surface marker. Two sub-populations of CD4+ cells, the Th1 and the Th2 cells, have been defined by in vitro cloning of T cells. They can be differentiated on the basis of the cytokines which they produce, and which determine their function. Th1 cells are involved in induction of cell-mediated immune responses. Th2 cells are involved in facilitating antibody production, especially IgE antibodies.

B cells mature into plasma cells and are responsible for producing antibody. Plasma cells responsible for IgE production are preferentially located in lymphoid tissue around the pharynx and under mucosal surfaces, sites where allergens gain access to the body. Their specificity for antigen remains unchanged throughout their lives, but the immunoglobulin isotype changes as the cell matures, from IgD and IgM to IgG, A or E. This is achieved by splicing out fragments of the DNA and linking various genes. Maturation

FIGURE 26.1 **Heterogeneity of CD4+ helper/inducer T cells distinguished by cytokine profile and function.**

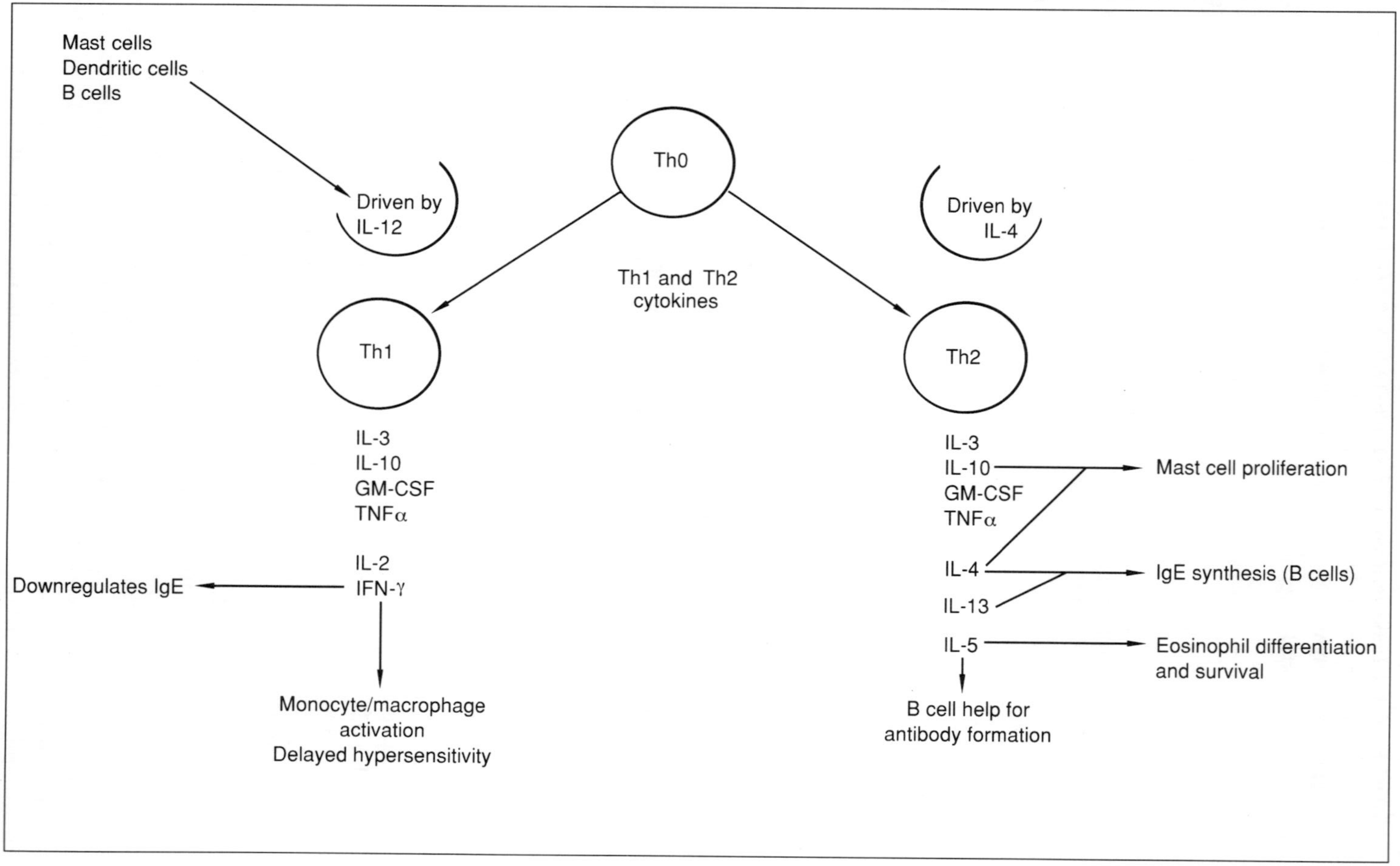

of B cells into the IgE-producing phenotype is favoured by IL4 and IL13, and down-regulated by interferon gamma. Since these are the cytokines produced by Th2 cells, preferential maturation of Th2 cells favours IgE production.

Mast cells are derived from progenitor stem cells in bone marrow. In many respects they resemble basophils, but they are derived from a distinct cell lineage, and as will be seen below, there are differences in their mediator profile. These cells play a central role in the allergic response by producing a variety of potent biological substances which have profound effects on tissues, and which also direct the immune response. Mast cells have functions outside

FIGURE 26.2 **Origin and some characteristics of mast cells and basophils.**

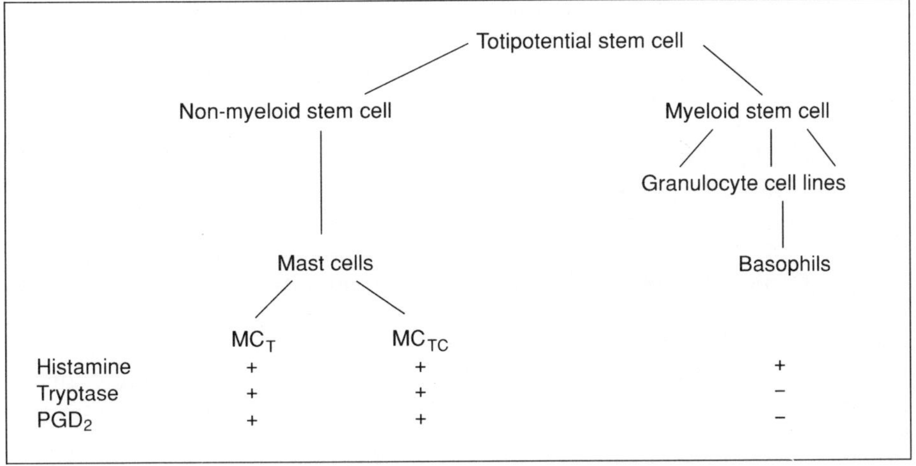

TABLE 26.2 **Heterogeneity of mast cells**

	MC_T	MC_{TC}
Synonym	Mucosal MC	Connective tissue MC
Distribution	Lung, especially alveoli Small intestinal mucosa Nasal mucosa	Submucosa of intestine Dermis, synovium Nasal mucosa
Histamine	+	+
Neutral proteases	Tryptase	Tryptase Chymase Carboxypeptidase Cathepsin G-like protease
Mediator production	PGD_2, LTC_4	PGD_2
Cytokine profile		
IL-4	+	+
TNFα	+	+
T cell dependency	Yes	No

of the allergic reaction, but these will not be considered further in this discussion. There are two types of mast cells previously known as connective tissue and mucosal mast cells (MC), but now described in accordance with their protease content as MC_{TC} and MC_T. They differ in the morphology of their granules, in their protease content, and their T cell dependence. Both have high affinity receptors for IgE ($FC_\varepsilon RI$) on their surface. Confusion has arisen in the past in distinguishing between these two populations because findings in mice and rats were extrapolated to humans, and it is now clear that these populations behave differently in various species. Their tissue distribution in humans is not as exclusive as in other species, and both types of mast cells are found together although in different proportions in different locations.

MC and basophils are the source of mediators of the allergic reaction. Their granules release preformed mediators, while from their phospholipid membranes are produced lipid mediators, the leukotrienes, prostaglandins and platelet-activating factor. They also produce cytokines which have profound effects on cell metabolism and potentiate further IgE production, and influence mast cell and eosinophil function. Basophils are present in the peripheral blood in very low numbers. However, they are present between the epithelial cells and in the mucus overlying the epithelial surfaces, and are therefore the first cells with which allergen comes in contact.

Eosinophils are derived from bone marrow precursors, and their production and activation is dependent on cytokines produced by T cells and mast cells. They are attracted to sites of allergic inflammation, where their release of highly potent enzymes leads to denudation of mucosal cells from the basement membrane and inflammation.

Neutrophils and macrophages also are attracted to sites of allergic inflammation and add to the inflammatory process by release of cytolytic enzymes and cytokines.

Vascular endothelium plays an active role in allergic inflammation by a number of mechanisms. These include release of adhesion molecules which allow inflammatory cells to attach and then leave the intravascular space en route to the inflammatory sites in the tissues. They allow the blood vessels to become more permeable and facilitate exudation of fluid.

Soluble agents

Immunoglobulin E. Since the 1920s it has been known that a serum factor was responsible for transfer of skin reactivity to allergen from one individual to another. This mysterious agent was known as a 'reagin', although its identity was not established until 1966 when a new class of antibody was described by Johansson and Bennich, and characterised by the Ishizaka husband and wife team. One reason that it took so long for IgE to be discovered is the minute amounts in serum, which required new technology to detect. IgE is similar in structure to other immunoglobulin molecules. It consists of two heavy and two light chains linked by disulphide bonds. Heavy chains are epsilon, light chains are kappa or lambda. However, it has an extra heavy chain domain and a higher content of sugars (glycosylation). IgE has evolved as a host defence mechanism against parasites. Parasitic infesta-

FIGURE 26.3 **The central role of mast cells in the allergic response.**

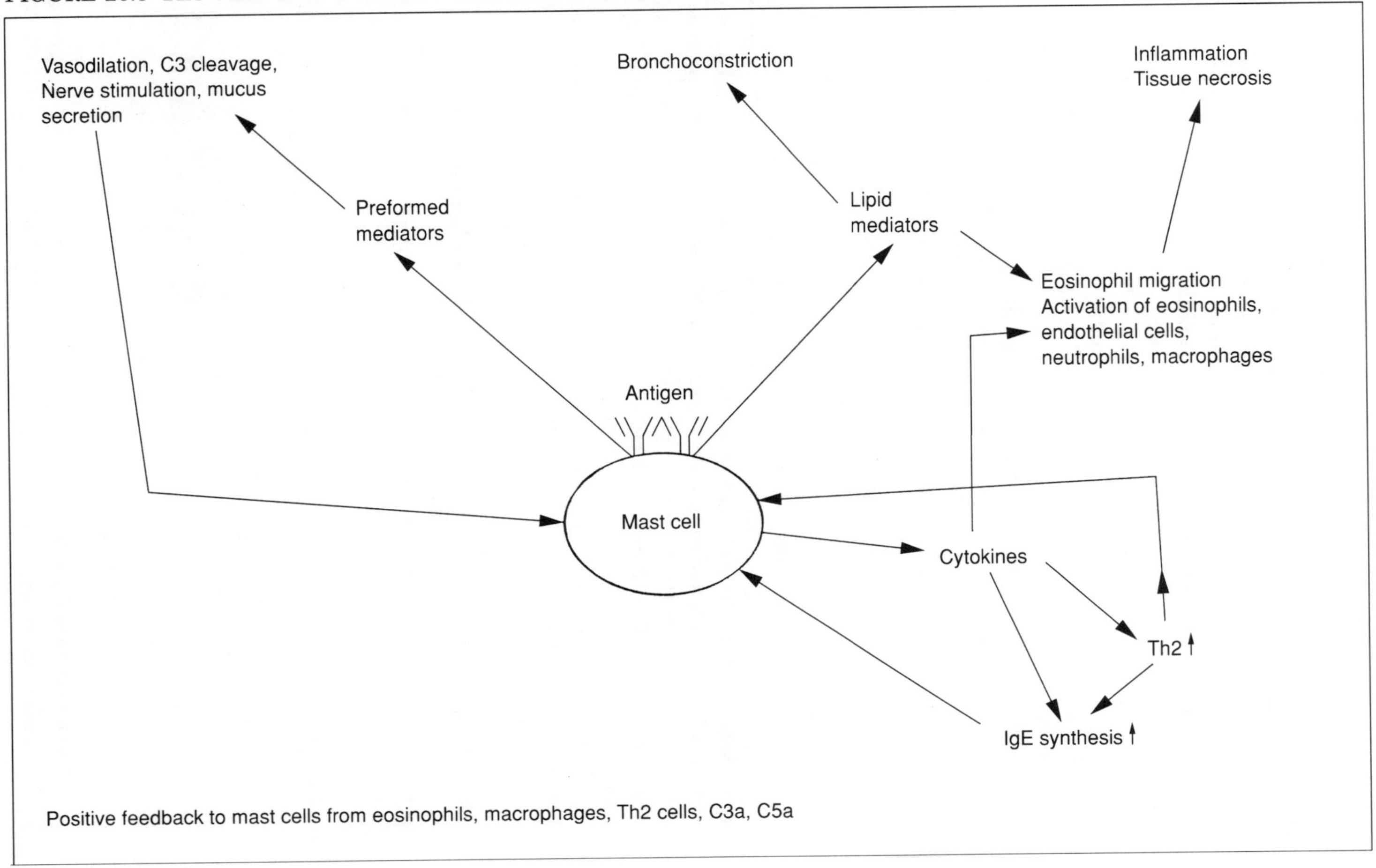

tion stimulates large amounts of non-specific IgE which may down-regulate specific IgE to allergens and thereby may explain why allergic diseases are phenomena of modern, developed countries.

The high affinity receptor for IgE on mast cells and basophils is termed Fc$_\varepsilon$RI. It has been sequenced, and consists of an α, a β and two γ chains. Recent work has shown it to be present also on Langerhans cells in the skin, an important antigen presenting cell population, on dendritic cells in the submucosa and on monocytes in atopics, especially those with atopic eczema. A low affinity IgE receptor (Fc$_\varepsilon$RII) has been described on other cells, including eosinophils, B cells and macrophages. Its function is not fully elucidated. However, it plays a role in cell activation and regulation of IgE production.

Other immunoglobulins. IgG4 is one of the subclasses of IgG which is present in low concentrations in serum. Its role in man is not clear. Increased serum levels follow desensitisation injections with bee venom, and high levels are found in bee-keepers In this context some authors feel it may be protective.

Mediators are molecules released by mast cells and basophils which execute the effects of the allergic reaction on target tissues. Some mediators are preformed and stored in granules, while others are newly formed as a result of lipid metabolism via the arachidonic acid pathway. These are the primary mediators. They act on other cells with release of secondary mediators. Release of preformed mediators stored in mast cell granules takes place within 1 to 5 minutes of antigen presentation. The energy for this process is provided by the adenylate cyclase pathway. Release of lipid mediators takes place over 5 to 30 minutes, and cytokine production follows in minutes to hours.

Histamine increases vascular permeability, causes smooth muscle contraction, and stimulates sensory nerve endings producing stinging and itch-

FIGURE 26.4 **Structure of immunoglobulin E and high affinity IgE receptor (FC$_\varepsilon$RI).**

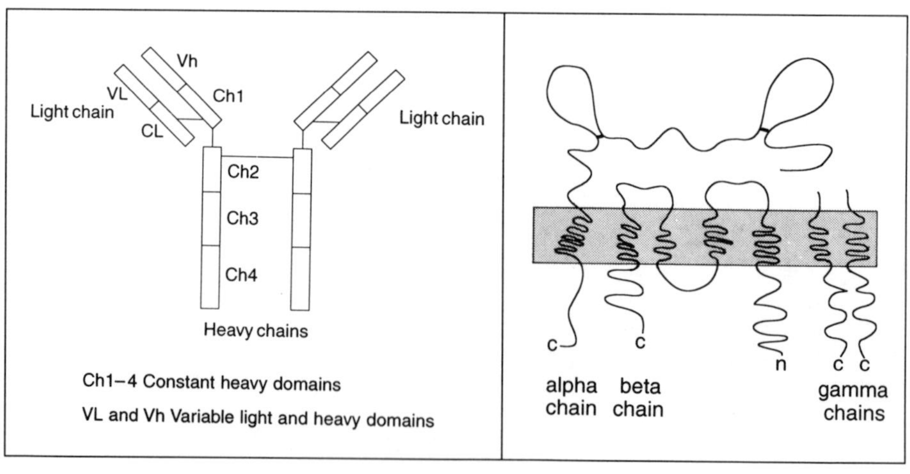

FIGURE 26.5 **Biochemical events in mediator release.**

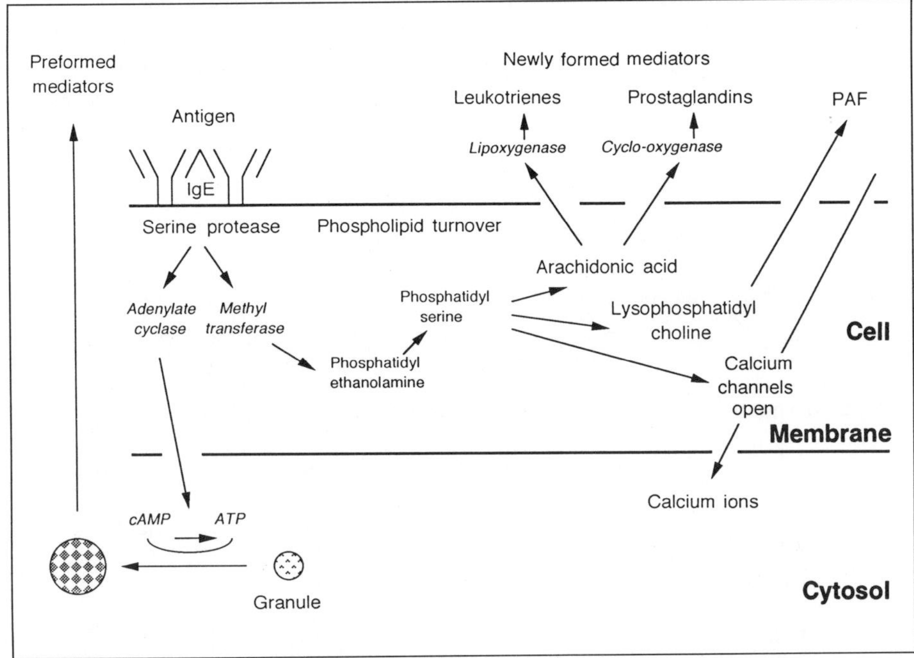

Table 26.3 **Mast cell mediators**

Preformed mediators
   Histamine
   Neutral proteases
      Tryptase
      Chymase
      Carboxypeptidase
   Chemotactic factors
      Eosinophil chemotactic factor (ECF)
      Neutrophil chemotactic factor (NCF)
   Acid hydrolases
   Oxidative enzymes

Newly generated mediators
   Prostaglandins
   Leukotrienes
   Platelet activating factor

Cytokines
   IL-4
   IL-5
   IL-6
   TNFα

FIGURE 26.6 **Biochemical events involved in formation of lipid mediators (eicosanoids, arachidonic acid pathway).**

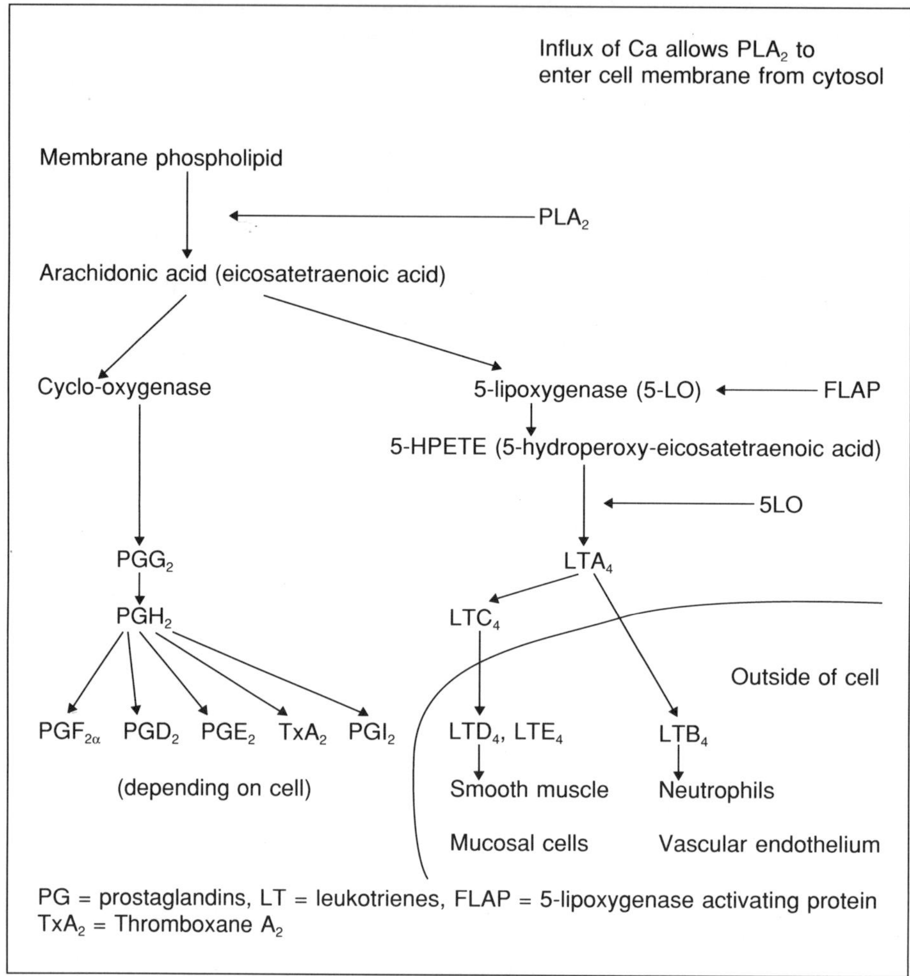

ing sensations and leading to production of neuropeptides which increase mast cell degranulation and enhance vascular permeability.

Tryptase is a protease found in secretory granules of mast cells but not basophils, thereby serving as a useful marker of mast cell activation. It contributes to the anticoagulant effects of heparin secreted by mast cells in the micro-environment, and causes fibrinolysis and cleavage of complement component C3. This latter increases mast cell activation.

Eosinophil chemotactic factor of anaphylaxis (ECF-A) is a chemokine secreted by mast cells which recruits eosinophils to the sites of allergic inflammation.

Cytokines are peptide molecules which act as messengers between a number of different cell types. They are produced by a variety of cells including T cells, mast cells, eosinophils, endothelial cells, macrophages and monocytes.When secreted by lymphocytes they are termed 'lymphokines'; when secreted by macrophages they are called 'monokines'; and lymphokines secreted by T cells are termed 'interleukins'. These messenger molecules have profound effects on the immune response. The same molecule often has different effects on different cell types. They may have multiple effects on one cell type. And different cytokines may have the same effect, leading to built-in redundancy. Cytokines can influence the effects of other cytokines, through antagonism or synergism. The net result of cytokine activity depends on an interaction of many agents, in what is effectively a 'cytokine network'. Cytokines include growth factors, induce differentiation, are chemotactic, pro-inflammatory and inhibitory. Two functional groups of CD4+ T helper cells can be distinguished on the profile of their cytokine production into Th1 and Th2 types with major implications for the pathogenesis of allergic diseases.

Adhesion molecules are surface membrane molecules which are actively involved in cell-to-cell interaction and are vital for all aspects of leucocyte function. These include activation of cells, homing of lymphocytes to appropriate tissue sites, maintenance of the viability of leucocytes in tissues, and chemotaxis. Cytokines increase or up-regulate the expression of adhesion molecules on cells, thereby enhancing the reactions between them. The inflammatory process depends on the exit of cells from blood vessels across the

TABLE 26.4 **Some cytokines and their biological functions**

Mediators of natural immunity
    Interferon α and β (IFNα, IFNβ)
    Tumour necrosis factor (TNF)
    IL-1
    IL-6

Chemotactic factors (chemokines)
    IL-8
    RANTES

Mediators of lymphocyte differentiation, growth and activation
    IL-2
    IL-4
    Transforming growth factor β (TGFβ)

Mediators of immune reactions
    IFNγ
    IL-5
    IL-10
    IL-12

Cell growth factors
    Granulocyte-macrophage colony stimulating factor (GM-CSF)
    Stem cell factor (c-kit ligand)
    IL-3
    IL-5
    IL-10
    Erythropoietin

TABLE 26.5 **Cell adhesion molecules**

Family	Molecule	Structure	Function	Distribution	Ligand
Integrins		α and β chains	Strong binding to cell adhesion molecules and extra cellular matrix		
β1				Lymphocytes	Fibronectin, matrix components
	VLA-4			Lymphocytes, monocytes	VCAM-1, Fibronectin
β2	LFA-1			Lymphocytes	ICAM-1, ICAM-2
	Mac-1			Macrophages	ICAM-1, iC3b
Selectins			Bind carbohydrates Initiate leucocyte-EC interaction		
	L-selectin			Leucocytes	ECs
	E-selectin (ELAM-1)			Cytokine activated EC	Sialyl Lewis x
	P-selectin			Cytokine activated EC	Sialyl Lewis x
Ig Superfamily		Single chain with homology to Ig	Cell adhesion Target for integrins		
	ICAM-1			ECs	LFA-1
	ICAM-2			ECs	LFA-1
	VCAM-1			Activated ECs	VLA-4
	CD2			T cells	LFA-3
	LFA-3			Lymphocytes	CD2
				APCs	

EC = endothelial cell
APC = antigen presenting cell

extravascular space to the site of inflammation and these processes depend on adhesion molecules. Cell adhesion molecules (CAM) are classified into three main groups.

1. *Integrins* are made up of non-covalently linked heavy (α) and light (β) chains on the surface of leucocytes. They are involved in adhesion of cells to matrix constituents including fibronectin and vitronectin, and to other cell types.
2. *Selectins* are a group of single chain glycoproteins present on leucocytes and endothelial cells.
3. *Immunoglobulin* superfamily molecules include intercellular adhesion molecules 1 and 2 (ICAM-1 and ICAM-2) and vascular cell adhesion molecule 1 (VCAM-1). They are single chain glycoproteins with considerable sequence homology to immunoglobulin-like domains. They are present on a variety of cells, including endothelial cells where they act as receptors for leucocyte integrins.

l-arginine—nitric oxide (NO) pathways

Identification of the endothelium derived relaxation factor as nitric oxide (NO) has led to a realisation that mammalian cells generate NO from l-arginine by a family of enzymes, the nitric oxide synthetases (NOS). Of these, nNOS (NOS I) and ecNOS (NOS III) are constitutive enzymes, found in neurones and endothelial cells respectively, while iNOS (NOS II) is inducible and leads to smooth muscle relaxation. Its expression is increased in airways of asthmatic patients and it may play a role in inducing the inflammation in asthmatic airways by inhibiting Th1 cells, leading to an increase in Th2 cells with all its consequences. There is a great increase in NO excretion in the airways of asthmatics related to the late allergic reaction. It also plays a role in induction of hypotension in conditions such as septic shock.

The plot

The process of *sensitisation* is brought about when processed antigen is presented to T cells by professional antigen presenting cells, including macrophages, dendritic cells such as Langerhans cells in the skin or B cells, in association with MHC Class II antigens. Resident alveolar macrophages appear to have an important regulatory function in the lung where they reduce the T cell response to inhaled antigen by suppressing the antigen presenting properties of dendritic cells and by inhibiting T cell proliferation.

TABLE 26.6 **Some biological actions of nitric oxide**

Tissue/System	Regulation
Vascular endothelium	Vasodilator tone—regulation of blood pressure
Lungs	Bronchodilation
Platelets	Aggregation
Heart	Contractility
Immune system	Cytotoxicity, cell signalling, non-specific immunity

T cells are activated, induce maturation of B cells into antibody producing plasma cells, and recruit further T cells. Communication between cells is achieved through the cytokine network and through direct cell contact. Plasma cells secrete IgE, which becomes attached to $Fc_\varepsilon RI$ on mast cells and basophils.

The next time the subject comes into contact with the allergen, an altered immune or allergic response occurs. The allergen attaches to the Fab fragments of two adjacent IgE molecules specific for the allergen. This cross-linking triggers a series of biochemical events resulting in the release of mediators and cytokines which produce the allergic inflammatory response (see Figure 26.7).

The result of the allergic reaction is the production within minutes of a wheal and flare in the skin, bronchospasm, itching, sneezing and rhinorrhoea, and vasodilatation with hypotension. This is the immediate reaction due to release of histamine and other preformed mediators.

The early response resolves and is followed some hours later by the late allergic reaction. This is due to recruitment of inflammatory cells to the area by lipid mediators, and cytokines secreted by T cells and mast cells. Eosinophils are prominent and a major contributor to tissue damage and shedding of mucosal cells. Persistence of the inflammatory reaction leads to secondary changes, including thickening of basement membrane, laying down of fibrin and eventual scarring.

The target tissue affected by allergic inflammation becomes hyperresponsive to a variety of non-specific stimuli. It is characteristic of asthma and explains why many asthmatics develop bronchospasm when exposed to cold air or a respiratory infection. Hyperresponsiveness is also a feature of nasal and skin allergy.

Development of an allergic response to antigen is favoured by the route of immunisation, being more likely when antigen is introduced across mucous membranes or skin, and by low doses of antigen. The nature of the antigen is also important.

Atopy is the tendency to react to environmental antigens by producing an allergic response to them. There is clearly a genetic component to atopy which explains why 'it runs in families'. We are starting to have a better understanding of the mechanisms involved in atopy. We know, for example, that atopic subjects tend to react to antigen differently from non-atopic individuals. They produce IgE antibody responses due to preferential upregulation of Th2 cells, rather than cell-mediated responses which are driven by Th1 cells. Many theories have been advanced for development of atopy, including the experience of heavy allergen loads early in life when the immune system is immature. At least 40% of the population is atopic, but only a proportion of this group develop clinically relevant disease.

Genetics of allergic diseases

It is well recognised that there is a familial clustering of allergic disease. The risk of allergy in a child increases with allergy in the parents. The prevalence of allergic disease of children where neither parent is allergic is

FIGURE 26.7 **Biology of IgE mediated immediate allergic reaction.**

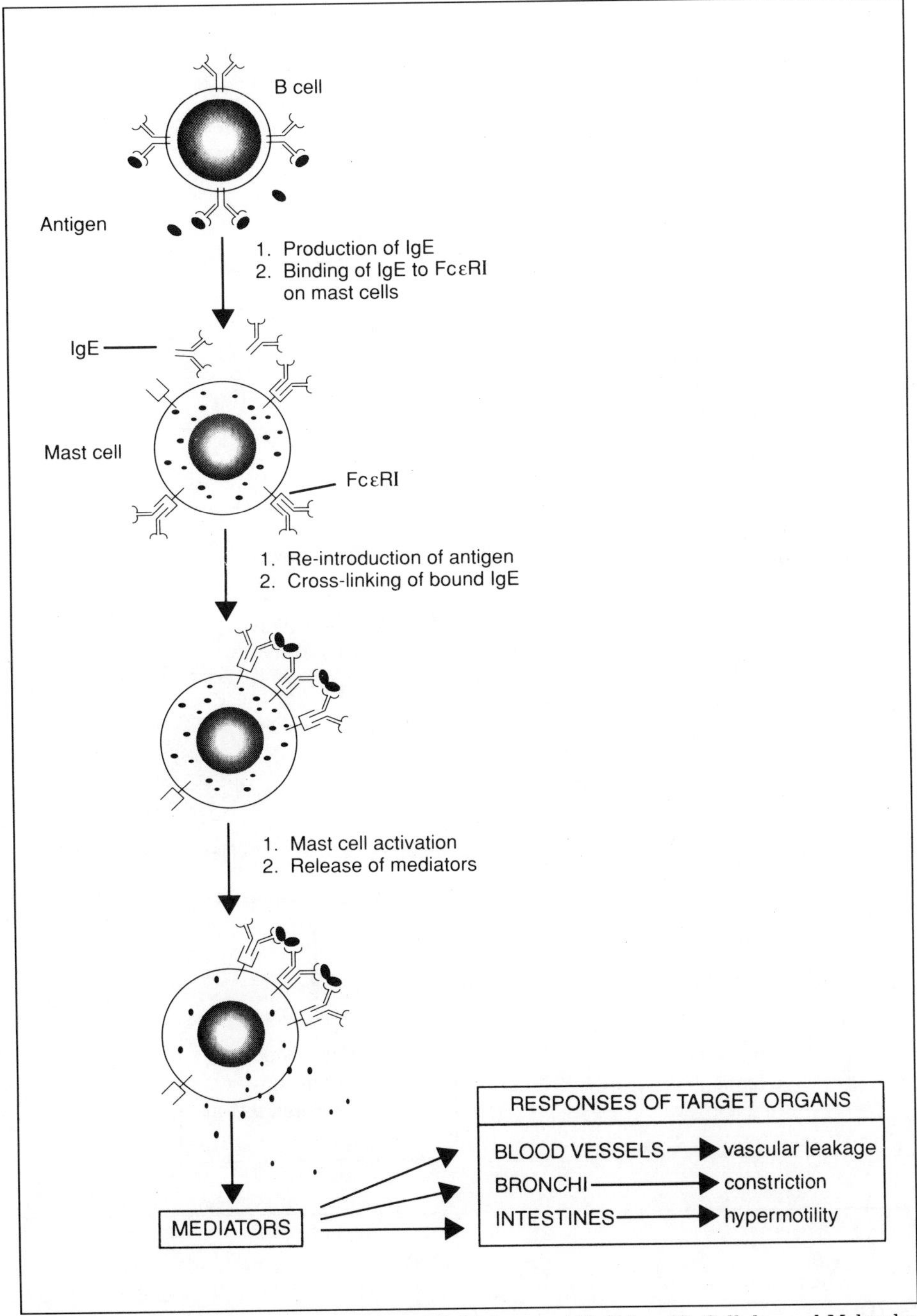

(Reproduced with permission from Abbas AK, Lightman AH, Pober JS. Cellular and Molecular Immunology. Philadelphia: WB Saunders, 1991).

FIGURE 26.8 **Biology of the late allergic reaction.**

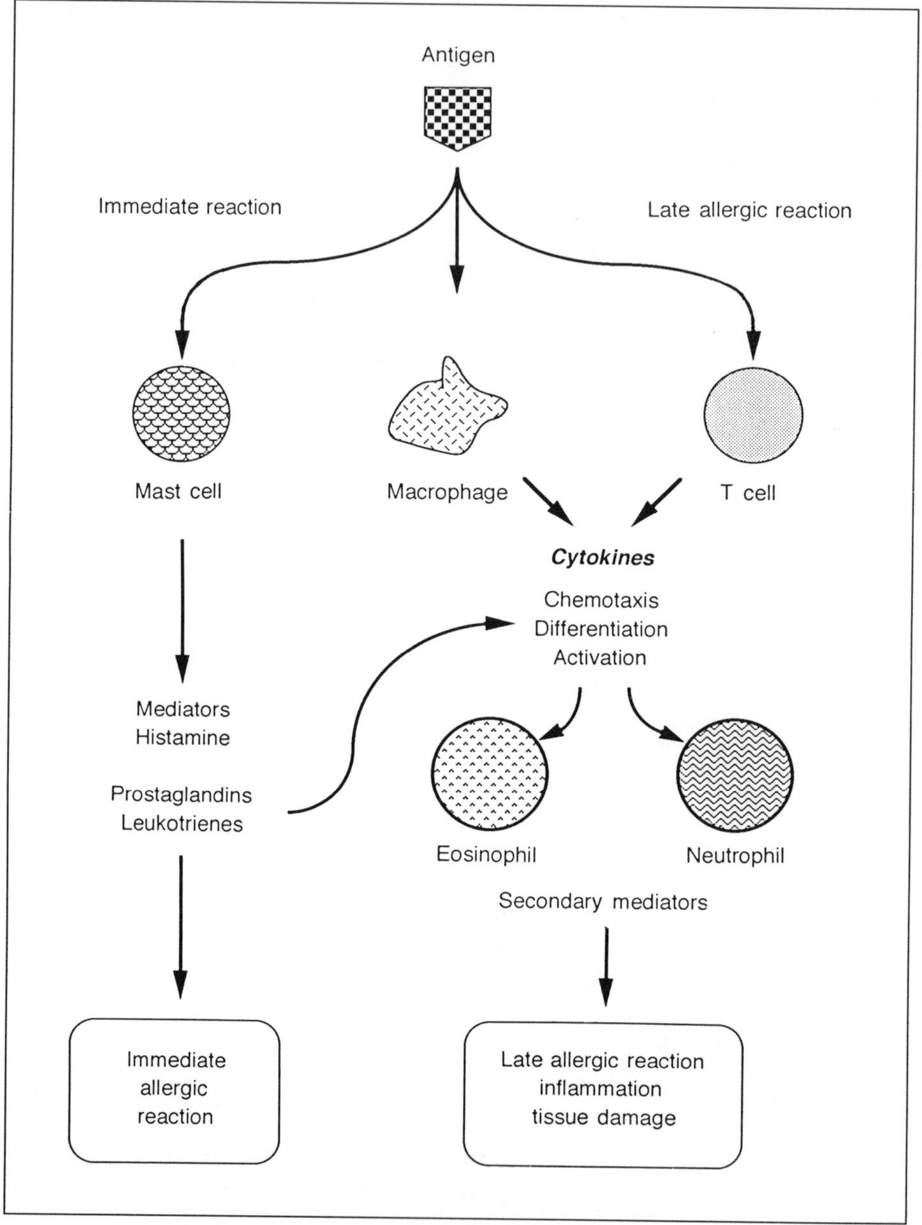

12%, where one parent is allergic is 45%, and where both parents are allergic is 70%.

Despite a large research effort, the genetics of these diseases is still the subject of much debate. Clearly the presence of allergy is not determined by a single locus. Unilocular inherited disorders are relatively rare in contrast to the complicated multigenic diseases such as asthma and allergy where genetic factors play a potential role at several levels. These include the tendency to sensitisation or atopy, the susceptibility of target tissues such as bronchial mucosa to react to stimuli, and immunological reactivity to specific allergens. Genetic studies need to take account of the fact that atopy can be present without symptoms if, for example, the opportunity for exposure to allergens is missing, and occasionally symptoms can be present without overt evidence of atopy.

Studies of the genetic basis of disease require three approaches. First, it is necessary to define the disease accurately in terms of its phenotype. This can be done on the basis of its pathology if diagnostic features are present, or functionally through physiological or immunological parameters. Unfortunately none of these criteria are unique to allergic disease, which makes phenotyping of allergic disease open to argument. Next, genetic analysis is applied using gene linkage studies and other techniques to define DNA polymorphisms which may be informative. Finally, molecular genetic techniques are used to map the genes and to clone and sequence them.

Specific antigen recognition is under genetic control, being determined by histocompatibility HLA-DR and T cell receptor antigens which are required for presentation of antigen and its interaction with antigen-sensitive cells. It is less clearly understood what determines the inheritance of the atopic trait. Some careful studies have suggested that atopy is dominantly inherited, determined by a single gene locus but with its expression depending on a host of other factors, both genetic and environmental. However, this is not widely accepted and other authorities favour a multiplicity of genes interacting at several levels. There must also be genetic influences on expression of the immunological reaction, for example determining bronchial hyper-responsiveness. Polymorphism of various receptors important in the allergic response have been described, such as the β2-adrenergic receptor and the high affinity IgE receptor, but it is still not clear what is the functional significance of these findings.

Allergens

Allergens are antigens which induce IgE mediated allergic reactions.

Properties of allergens

It is not clear what inherent properties make antigens become allergens. Most are glycoproteins, protein molecules with varying sugar content. Their molecular weights vary between 10 kD and 100 kD, with many around 40 kD. However, allergic responses can be stimulated by much smaller molecules when they function as haptens and are attached to carrier proteins such as skin proteins. A good example is nickel which is a common cause of contact dermatitis.

Classification and nomenclature

The individual allergens of most materials responsible for inducing allergic reactions have been identified by now and sequenced, and their amino acid structures are known. This is a major step forward in allergy since it allows the synthesis of highly purified allergens and fragments of allergens or peptides which can be used in diagnosis and therapy.

Allergens are described as major or minor, depending on whether more or less than 50% of patients have IgE antibodies to them. This nomenclature does not necessarily indicate the biological potency of the allergen.

To bring some order to the large number of allergens now recognised, a new allergen nomenclature has been adopted by the World Health Organiza-

TABLE 26.7 **Nomenclature of some common allergens**

Source of allergen	Allergens	Function	MW (kD)	Sequence data
Grass pollens				
Rye grass (*Lolium perenne*)	Lol p 1		27	C
	Lol p 2–3		11	C
	Lol p 5		31	P
	Lol p 9		31/35	C
Bermuda grass (*Cynodon dactylon*)	Cyn d 1		32	C
Tree pollens				
Birch (*Betula verrucosa*)	Bet v 1		17	C
	Bet v 2	profilin	15	C
Olive (*Olea europea*)	Ole e 1		16	C
Dust mites (*Dermatophagoides* sp):				
D. pteronyssinus	Der p 1	Cysteine protease	25	C
	Der p 2–7			
	Der p 3	Serine protease		
D. farinae	Der f 1	Cysteine protease	25	C
	Der f 2–3			
Animals				
Cat saliva (*Felis domesticus*)	Fel d 1		38	C
Moulds				
Alternaria alternata	Alt a 1		28	P
Insects				
Honey bee (*Apis mellifera*)	Api m 1	phospholipase A	16	C
	Api m 2	hyaluronidase	44	C
	Api m 4	mellitin	3	C
Wasp (*Polistes annularis*)	Pol a 1	phospholipase	35	P
Numerous other wasp species				
Foods and others				
Codfish (*Gadus callarias*)	Gad c 1		12	C

P = partial, C = complete.
(Adapted from King et al, 1995. The original article should be referred to for a full list of allergens and more details).

tion and International Union of Immunological Societies (WHO/IUIS). Allergens are assigned the first three letters of the genus, followed by the first letter of the species and a number indicating the order in which the allergens were first described. Additional letters are used in some instances to avoid ambiguities. Allergens from single species may consist of several similar molecules. These are known as isoallergens if they are of similar size, have identical biological function, and 67% or greater amino acid identity. Recombinant and synthetic peptides have the same nomenclature, but with the prefix *r* or *s* respectively. Other details may also appear such as the residue positions. Table 26.7 shows some examples of these allergens.

Specificity and cross-reactivity

Allergen recognition by the immune system is highly specific and is directed to small components of the molecules known as epitopes. It is possible for different epitopes of the same antigen to be recognised by different subjects. Epitopes may be shared between different allergens or there may be partial identity. This is more likely to be the case between related species.

A high degree of cross-reactivity can be seen between some plant species and this is due to the presence of profilins which function as common antigens for a variety of species. *Profilins* are proteins of molecular weight 12–16 kD which are present in all eukaryotic cells. They bind to actin, to membrane phospholipids and to proline rich sequences of proteins, and they are involved in a number of vital cellular motility functions. Although not major allergens in any plant species, reactivity to them could explain the multiple sensitivities of many allergic patients to pollens from a wide range of unrelated species. It has been estimated that about 20% of pollen-allergic patients react with profilin.

Further reading

Immunology

Barnes PJ, Liew FY. Nitric oxide and asthmatic inflammation. *Immunol Today* 1995; 16: 128–30.

Bradding P. Human mast cell cytokines. *Clin exp Allergy* 1996; 26: 13–19.

Canonica GW, Ciprandi G, Buscaglia S, Pesce G, Bagnasco M. Adhesion molecules of allergic inflammation: recent insights into their functional roles. *Allergy* 1994; 49: 135–41.

Holt PG, Sedgwick JD. Suppression of IgE responses following antigen inhalation: a natural homeostatic mechanism which limits sensitisation to aeroallergens. *Immunology Today* 1987; 8: 14.

Holt PG. Allergen presentation in the airways. *In:* Johansson SGO (ed). Progress in Allergy and Clinical Immunology. Seattle: Hogrefe and Huber, 1995; 3: 1–4.

Moncado S, Higgs A. The 1-arginine–nitric oxide pathway. *New Engl J Med* 1993; 329: 2002–12.

Romagnani S, Del Prete GF, Maggi E, Ricci M. TH1 and TH2 cells and their role in disease. *Allergy Clin Immunol News* 1993; 5: 19–22.

Genetics

Bleeker ER, Meyers DA. Recent advances in the genetics of asthma. *Clin exp Allergy* 1995; 25 Suppl 2: 1–2.

Allergens

King TP, Hoffman D, Lowenstein H, Marsh DG, Platts-Mills TAE, Thomas W. Allergen nomenclature. World Health Organization/IUIS Allergen Nomenclature Subcommittee. *J Allergy Clin Immunol* 1995; 96: 5–14.

Knox B, Suphioglu C. Environmental and molecular biology of pollen allergens. *Trends in Plant Science* 1996; 1: 156–64.

Chapter 27

Aerobiology

Aerobiology is the study of airborne particles, quality of air, and distribution and behaviour of particles. A knowledge of the principles of aerobiology is necessary for understanding the epidemiology of allergic diseases. It also contributes significantly to the proper management of these diseases in individual patients by providing accurate information about the most important allergens in particular geographic areas and at particular times of year. It predicts what conditions are likely to give rise to most problems and indicates preventative steps which can ameliorate clinical effects. Determination of climatic variables such as the presence of inverse weather conditions and prevailing winds can explain distribution of airborne particles and allergens.

The most important *outdoor allergens* are pollens, sub-microscopic particulate matter which may arise from breakdown of intact pollen grains, and mould spores. The prevalence of these allergens is regional and seasonal and depends on atmospheric conditions. They are difficult to avoid.

The most important *indoor airborne allergens* are house dust mite faecal pellets, components of insects such as cockroach, cat and other animal danders, and mould spores. These materials are prevalent throughout the year, their presence depends to some degree on human activity and they are therefore controllable. Morphologically they are difficult to identify.

Pollens are generally not found to any great extent indoors, but this depends on living habits. Indoor pollen counts are low where air-conditioning is in common usage or windows are kept closed. However, where cooling is achieved by air circulation through the house such as occurs in traditional Queensland homes, pollen counts can be high within the house.

Most airborne allergens are from 5–60 microns in size. Particles greater than 18–20 microns are excluded from entry to the airways below the carina, whereas particles less than 5 microns can enter and remain beyond the terminal bronchioles. This raises the question of how sensitisation and provocation of symptoms occur in asthma. Possible explanations are the stimulation of reflexes by particles in upper airways, or the presence of submicronic fragments of pollens and other allergens which gain access to lungs. The presence of such material has been confirmed.

Where several different pollen species appear sequentially, the earlier ones may prime the patient so that their reaction to the later allergens will be enhanced. For example, it was found that a heavy flowering season for Paterson's Curse in the Riverina was followed by a more severe grass pollen season.

External environment

The distribution of external environmental allergens can be measured by various collection devices. These work by directing a stream of air over or on to a sticky surface so that the particulate matter remains on the surface and can be identified. A wide range of collection devices is available for particular requirements, for example to enable sampling of indoor environments. Volumetric devices sample measured volumes of air, thereby providing a quantitative guide to the amount of material present. If such collections are timed, pollen profiles can be established for various time periods. One of the most useful of these devices is the Burkard Pollen Counter (Figure 27.1) which has a rotating drum with an adhesive coated strip on to which is directed a stream of air at 10 L/min. At the end of 7 days the strip is removed, fixed, stained and examined. Pollen identification and counting is time-consuming and requires considerable expertise. Immunochemical techniques relying on monoclonal antibodies and molecular biology are being developed which will make the procedure more efficient.

Pollen grains

Pollen is the male gamete responsible for fertilising the female flower. This takes place in one of two ways. With perfumed, highly conspicuous and

FIGURE 27.1 **A Burkard 7 day pollen counter on top of a tall building.** The vane directs the orifice in the direction of the prevailing wind while a small electric pump directs a stream of air on to an adhesive strip on a rotating drum within the machine.

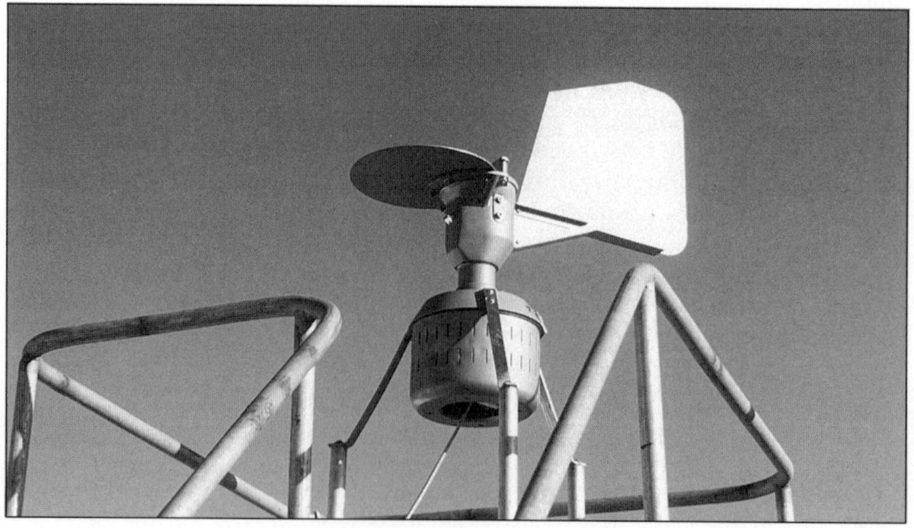

brightly coloured flowers, pollination is dependent on insects which are attracted to the glamour of the flower and brush against the male anther. Some pollen sticks to the body of the insect and is transferred to the stamen when it visits a female flower. *Insect-pollinated* plants produce sticky pollen in low amounts and are usually not responsible for pollinosis—they are termed '*entomophilous*' plants.

The other method of pollenation depends on the production of vast amounts of pollen which are dispersed in prevailing winds. These *anemophilous or wind-pollinated* species are the major culprits in respiratory allergy. Entomophilous species often get blamed for producing allergic symptoms since their brightly coloured flowers make a show at the same time as the pollenation of the inconspicuous wind-pollenated plants. Exceptions do occur. With heavy crops of insect-pollenated plants, sufficient amounts of pollen may be produced for it to be found in the atmosphere and to be responsible for induction of allergy. A good example are the stands of Paterson's Curse which covered the landscape in the Riverina areas of New South Wales and Victoria, and could be shown to cause sensitisation and symptoms. Biological control methods have reduced numbers of these plants. Privet and wattle are insect-pollenated but their pollens can lead to sensitisation when people remain in close proximity to the plants.

The distribution of pollens is highly dependent on geographical and climatic factors which affect the growth of plants and the production and distribution of pollens. Grasses are the major sources of pollen in Australia, with a contribution from weeds and trees. Flora introduced into Australia are the most troublesome sources of allergenic pollen. Native species are not major sources of allergen, with a few exceptions such as Callitris pine in rural New South Wales and in Queensland. Problems are not described with the eucalypts. Melaleuca species give infrequent skin responses, especially in the

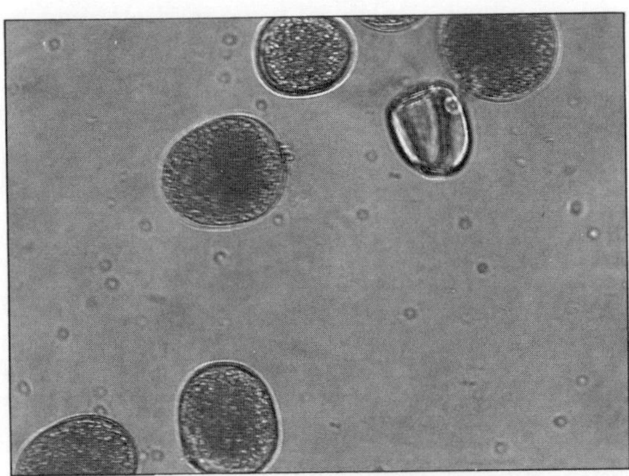
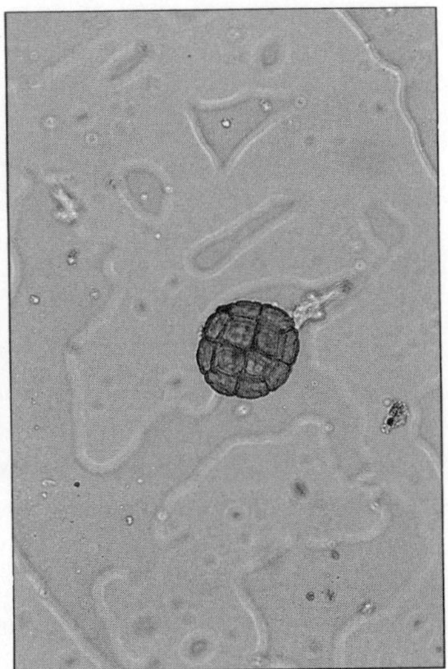

FIGURE 27.2 **Pollen grains.** (a) Rye grass is an anemophilous or wind-pollinated species, and (b) wattle is a sticky pollen which is entomophilous or insect-pollinated.
(Photomicrographs kindly supplied by Dr D. Bass).

city, as does casuarina (she-oak). Acacia (wattle) is the second most prolific genus after eucalypts in Australia and pollination seasons of different species extend throughout most of the year. Wattle pollens are heavy and do not travel far. They can produce symptoms, although some degree of cross-reactivity with rye grass pollen has been reported.

The conditions favouring pollinosis are hot, dry windy weather, lawn-mowing, travelling through areas of heavy pollination and being outdoors. Rain washes pollens out of the atmosphere, resulting in improvement of symptoms. Pollen-induced disease is also better in cooler weather, at the beach and indoors, especially in air-conditioned environments.

Micro-environmental distribution of pollens relates to the presence of pollens in a small area and this depends on local plantings, as well as the results of wind-borne pollens from a distance. Heavy plantings of plants, which may not normally depend on wind pollination, may result in heavy atmospheric loads of pollens, for example Paterson's Curse in the Riverina, plane trees in Sydney, elms in Melbourne and local ferns and tree ferns which sporulate in January. At an even more local level, garden plantings can influence the immediate vicinity. This aspect has tended to be ignored but is important as it is amenable to modification.

Fungal spores

These are difficult to study because of the variability in morphology even within the same species, depending on the phase of growth. Little is known about the behaviour of the different species.

Inorganic particulate matter

Over recent years there has been an increasing realisation of the importance of particulate matter and pollution in causing respiratory allergies. Inorganic particles, especially aluminosilicates, may be responsible for some of the manifestations of asthma, possibly by acting as adjuvants which stimulate the immune response or as carriers of allergens. Diesel fume particles can be shown to be immune stimulants, at least in vitro. More recently it has become recognised that latex particles originating from motor vehicle tyres are present in urban air samples and may be important factors in latex sensitisation, as well as in acting as adjuvants and facilitating sensitisation to other allergens.

Indoor environment

The indoor environment is being more closely studied now as a result of the epidemic of house dust mite allergy which followed the energy crisis in the 1970s when houses in Denmark in particular were built sealed as far as possible to avoid loss of heat to the environment and to reduce heating costs. This increased the indoor humidity, thereby rendering the ecoclimate more favourable for house dust mites and increasing their rate of reproduction.

House dust mites are the major indoor allergens. The faecal pellets are 5 microns in diameter. Because of their size, they remain suspended in the air for long periods after dust is disturbed and therefore are easily inspired into the lungs. Other important allergens are cat dander and cockroach. Inner city suburbs are more likely to be plagued by the latter, and more affluent populations by cats. Other components include fungal spores, especially alternaria which is a dry climate aeroallergen.

Role of aerobiology in clinical practice

Maps showing the distribution of pollens are valuable in defining which allergens are likely to be clinically relevant in particular areas and assist in selecting appropriate allergens for skin testing and in preparation of extracts for immunotherapy. One example of their value was the recent demonstration that couch (Bermuda) grass pollen is an important allergen in Alice Springs, an arid, semi-desert area.

The timing and duration of pollination varies with geographical and climatic conditions and this determines the onset and duration of symptoms. The grass pollen season is prolonged in warmer climates and in some areas may persist for most of the year. In colder areas the season is much shorter and may start as late as November.

Pollen counting may help to explain various epidemics of respiratory allergy by demonstrating peak of allergens coinciding with major outbreaks of symptoms in the population. Some weather patterns lead to accumulation of pollens and respiratory allergies may then follow. For example, an outbreak of asthma in Tamworth in 1990 coincided with thunderstorm activity following several days of hot weather, at the time that rye grass was flowering in the surrounding districts.

The predictive value of aerobiology is much less certain. Some weather conditions are conducive to high levels of pollution, particulate matter or pollens, but the limitations of this procedure are similar to those of weather forecasting. Daily pollen count data are usually available only in retrospect and hence of limited value for the individual patient.

Specific prevalence data

Pollen maps have been prepared for various areas of Australia and are continuing to be developed. Data available for major geographical areas is summarised below.

Major Australian cities and regions

Sydney and New South Wales. The distribution of aeroallergens is different in various regions of the city. House dust mite is the predominant allergen, especially in the inner and eastern suburbs, while grass pollens are more prominent towards the west and the north-west. *Parietaria judaica* (wall pellitory), a Mediterranean weed, has spread throughout the metropolitan area from its original distribution on the lower North Shore to other areas and has now been sighted in most other areas of Sydney. Its pollen is found more at ground level so that it is often a more localised problem affecting particular houses or streets. It produces symptoms from September to March with a second peak in February. Important tree species are plane trees, which pollenate in early September, and privet. The small-leaved privet

(Ligustrum sinense) cross-reacts with the olive tree and pollinates from September through October and its pollen cross-reacts antigenically with that of the olive tree. The big-leaved variety *(Ligustrum lucidum)* pollinates from late December to February.

On the Western Slopes which are less humid than coastal areas, alternaria is the predominant allergen for asthma. In other parts of rural New South Wales grass pollens are the predominant allergens. Other troublesome species are Callitris pine which pollinates from late July to mid-September, and Monterey pine *(Cupressus macrocarpa)* which pollinates from July to August.

Melbourne. The seasons are well-defined. Trees pollenate in late winter and early spring, the predominant species being elm and cypress, accounting for more than 90% of the pollen in winter, while tree pollens account for over 60% of total pollens during the rest of the year. Elms are widely planted in public spaces in Melbourne. Grasses then follow in spring, the predominant species being rye and canary grasses, both introduced as pasture grasses. Various weeds and herbs are found later in the year. There is a minor peak of olive and privet pollen in October and November, although these are predominantly insect-pollenated species.

Canberra is notorious for grass pollen allergy. However, there have been extensive plantings of exotic European trees such as birch, ash, maple, cypress and oak which are prolific pollinators. The tree pollination season starts in August and lasts until the end of October, whereas grasses start pollinating in early October, peak in November, and continue at a high level until the end of December.

Brisbane and Queensland. House dust mite is the major aeroallergen in Brisbane. Grass pollens are perennial allergens as there is a prolonged grass pollination season extending from September to May, including some winter pollination. The predominant species are couch, sorghum (Johnson) and paspalum. Owing to the open ventilation of the houses, grass pollens are also present indoors.

Trees are not a major problem in Queensland, but an important species is the Bribie Island or Murray pine (Callitris species) which is distributed particularly around Hervey Bay and Roma. Little is known about Melaleuca species. Weed pollens occur in regional pockets of Queensland. Ragweed (Artemisia species) is found in the Tweed Heads area of northern New South Wales and pollinates in autumn. The season lasts 4 to 5 weeks and few patients are severely affected. Plantain is common in the Darling Downs, while parthenium, which was imported from India and Mexico and is related to ragweed, is found in central Queensland, north-west of Toowoomba. It flowers in late summer. It causes a contact dermatitis but the lack of suitable reagents precludes extensive skin testing to determine its role in respiratory allergy.

In *Adelaide* seasonal allergy due to grass pollen is prevalent. However, olive trees have proliferated to weed proportions throughout the Adelaide Hills and are proving to be an increasing problem. Callitris (white cypress) is another common species of tree.

Perth. The grass pollen season is greatly extended, commencing in July with a peak in August, another peak in November and then persisting through to March, with another minor peak in that month. Of the allergenic trees, Cupressus and Callitris pollens are prevalent from August to October, and Prunus from late July to early November.

Hobart. With the colder temperatures in Hobart, the grass-pollinating season is shorter and most allergies occur between October and December. Plane trees (Plantanus species) are the important allergenic tree species.

Alice Springs. Couch grass *(Cynodon dactylon)* is the major aeroallergen and increases markedly after rain. At these times there is a significant increase in hospital admissions in the non-aboriginal population from asthma.

Cairns. House dust mite is the major allergen, but several grass species are important between October and December, and paspalum from January to May.

Darwin. No information is available.

Further applications of aerobiology

Since most of the heavily pollinating plants which are important clinically are introduced, a good case can be made for encouraging the planting of native pastures. A start has been made with the production of the seed of wallaby grass *(Danthonia)* and kangaroo grass *(Themada australis)*. The prolific pollination of introduced species probably is a major factor in their success, so it remains to be seen whether the low-pollinating native species will adequately serve the same purposes.

There is a similar rationale for replanting of denuded forests with natural species, and for encouraging the local planting of low-allergen species in gardens, streetscapes and open spaces. Even though grass pollens and other wind-borne pollens may travel great distances on wind currents, there are many examples of local problems arising from heavy planting, and this can relate even to predominantly insect-pollenated species. This is becoming recognised and some authorities are taking appropriate action to concentrate on native and low-pollenating species.

Further reading

Bass DA. The low allergen garden. *Modern Medicine* 1995; 38: 52–64.
Bass DA. Clinically important pollens of NSW and the ACT. *Med J Aust* 1984. Suppl.

Chapter 28

New promises for management of allergy

In the past decade our understanding of the basic mechanisms of allergy has expanded and we are now able to apply our knowledge to achieve a far more targeted approach to the management of allergic disease. So far we have had to rely on β-2 agonists and antihistamines to provide symptomatic relief, and on crude non-specific measures such as corticosteroids for reducing inflammation in affected tissues, and subcutaneous injection of allergens for deviating the immune response. These measures have made important contributions to the fundamental management of allergic disease but they are associated with considerable costs in terms of morbidity. We are now able to target specific events in the allergic response, for example diverting T cell development from Th2 to Th1 phenotype, using immunosuppressive agents, or inhibiting and antagonising specific enzymes, mediators and other biological measures in the immune process. In doing so we are also finding that a number of such measures have anti-inflammatory properties similar to those of corticosteroids without the potentially harmful effects of these drugs.

Modulating T cell function and cytokine profiles

The basic defect in allergic disease is a relative imbalance in cytokines, with deficiency of IFN-γ and excessive activity of IL-4. This leads to increased emphasis on Th2 production and function, and increased IgE production.

Immunotherapy with allergens corrects this defect by favouring the development of T cells with the Th1 cytokine profile by a variety of mechanisms, including the upregulation of IL-12. This approach has been limited by the inability to provide an adequate immunising dose because of the risk of initiating allergic reactions. Recent work has defined specific *T cell epitopes* of these allergens and has led to the ability to separate the immunogenic properties from the allergenic properties of these molecules. Immunisation with these T cell epitopes appears to modulate the late phase allergic reaction and possibly down-regulate histamine releasing factors. The ideal reagent is one which requires one or few injections, is of long duration, with no side effects and which is particularly not IgE fixing, and which is capable of switching the T cell cytokine profile from Th2 to Th1 cells. Peptides, which are being trialled to determine their clinical efficacy with a number of allergens such as house dust mite and cat, can be generated. Preliminary trials with cat allergens have been promising with improvement in bronchial challenge results 6 weeks after therapy. Immediate reactions have been rare but delayed reactions have occurred, possibly due to production of histamine releasing factors.

Cytokine therapy. In allergic disease the imbalance between IFN-γ and IL-4 favours production of T cells with the Th2 cytokine profile and isotype switching of B cells to IgE production. IFN-γ has been administered, therefore, in an attempt to correct this underlying defect and this has proved to be effective in some trials in atopic eczema. However, results in asthma have so far been equivocal. A recent experimental study by Gelfand's group (Lack G and Gelfand EW, *ACI International* 1996; 8: 30–3) suggests that the reasons for this lack of success are that the agent needs to be administered early, with allergen, and locally to the site of the tissue reaction. Such requirements could perhaps be met, at least partially, by IFN-γ administered by inhalation, and trials of such therapy will be awaited with much interest.

Interleukin 5 (IL-5) is an important cytokine which enhances eosinophil recruitment, maturation, survival and activation. Eosinophils play an important role in allergic inflammation, causing tissue destruction and stripping of epithelial cells. One action of glucocorticoids is to reduce the synthesis of IL-5, thereby contributing to their anti-inflammatory properties. However, efforts are being made to find more specific inhibitors of IL-5, one candidate being the production of humanised monoclonal anti-IL-5 antibody.

Immunosuppressives. Cyclosporin A has a specific effect on T cells and reduces numbers of Th2 phenotype cells in inflammatory sites. Several trials of its use in severe asthma have suggested that it is useful in reducing numbers of infiltrating Th2 cells and in ameliorating asthma in refractory severe cases, but, as with other immunosuppressives such as methotrexate, its role is far from established. It has also been used in atopic eczema with some success. Its long-term use is associated with serious side effects which limit its usefulness.

Mediators: inhibition of production and antagonism of action

Antihistamines are the classical mediator antagonists. They have been available for many years. However, newer drugs are being developed which are non-sedating and which are free of cardiac toxicity. Some of the newer agents have also been found to have other anti-allergy properties such as inhibiting adhesion molecules interacting with their ligands. The clinical significance of these other actions still needs to be established, but it has led many authors to suggest that the newer agents should no longer be considered as merely antihistamines but as anti-allergy drugs with antihistamine properties being but one of their functions.

Antagonists of other mediators have eluded clinical usefulness until recently. However, a number of candidate drugs have been investigated and several have reached clinical trial stage.

Phosphodiesterase inhibitors increase levels of cyclic adenosine monophosphate (cAMP) which with cyclic guanosine monophosphate (cGMP) are important second messengers in regulating mediator secretion and smooth muscle tone. Increased cAMP results in reduced mediator release with smooth muscle relaxation, and in the lungs, bronchodilation. Theophylline is the classical agent of this class. However, its therapeutic index is low and it is associated with significant side effects which do not justify its limited therapeutic potential. However, at least five distinct phosphodiesterase isoenzymes have been identified, and specific inhibitors are being developed. Phosphodiesterases are widely distributed, especially in the airway, in vascular smooth muscle and in inflammatory cells, and consequently they have a wide variety of properties. Inhibitors of a number of these isoenzymes have been developed. Many have unacceptable side effects, but inhibitors of PDE IV hold the promise of bronchodilation with potent anti-inflammatory properties and without the hypotension caused by vasodilation (since PDE IV is not found in vascular smooth muscle). Rolipram is a representative agent. PDE inhibitors have also been trialled topically in atopic eczema with good preliminary results. Topically they have the advantage of affecting a variety of inflammatory and immune pathways without the problem of systemic side effects.

Leukotriene inhibitors and antagonists. Research has advanced to the stage of identifying a number of substances which are effective in reducing the response to cold air, exercise and aspirin, and in the clinical treatment of asthma. Receptor antagonists include zafirlukast and pranlukast, and inhibitors of synthesis include zileuton and MK-0591, a FLAP (5-lipoxygenase activating protein) inhibitor. Side effects so far have been few and limited mainly to headache. Zafirlukast has been released in some overseas markets for prophylaxis of asthma in patients aged 12 years and over who are not adequately controlled on β-agonists which are used on an 'as required' basis. It needs to be administered on a regular daily basis. The exact clinical role of these agents still remains to be established. It is not yet clear whether they should be used in mild to moderate asthma or whether they should be restricted to the more severe cases. More clinical experience will be necessary for the whole picture to emerge and to address questions of cost-benefit analysis.

Tryptase inhibitors. Tryptase comprises 20% of the total protein in mast cells and it has been implicated in the pathogenesis of asthma, although this has been difficult to prove because of the lack of specific inhibitors. However, inhibitors such as APC 366, which reduce the early allergic reaction and block the late allergic reaction in experimental situations, are now being developed. Of great importance is the fact that tryptase appears to be anti-inflammatory, to reduce accumulation of eosinophils and to completely block airway hyperresponsiveness after allergen challenge.

Anti-adhesion molecule therapy

Cell adhesion molecules (CAM) play a vital role in the inflammatory response, allowing intravascular leucocytes to adhere to endothelium preparatory to leaving the circulation, and to migrate to tissue sites of inflammation where they are activated. Adhesion molecules play a role at all steps in this process. Interfering with their function can have potentially enormous biological effects, inhibiting inflammatory processes, not only in allergic diseases, but also in other situations such as tumour biology, graft rejection and thrombosis. There are several approaches to interfering with CAM function. Monoclonal antibodies can be raised to particular components. Antibody to ICAM-1 has shown some promise in primate models of airway inflammation. Interference with the interaction of selectins with the carbohydrate components of their ligands can be achieved with simple carbohydrates and other molecules such as low molecular weight heparin. Several peptide analogues such as Arg-Gly-Asp have been developed which block adhesion molecule function, and offer another potential therapeutic approach. It must be emphasised that these approaches are still experimental. There are several H1 antagonists and other agents already in clinical use which down-regulate ICAM-1 on epithelial cells, but the clinical importance of this function is not clear. These drugs include cetirizine, fexofenadine (TAM, the metabolite of terfenadine), levocabastine, loratidine, terfenadine, nedocromil, deflazacort and budesonide.

Nitric oxide synthetase (NOS) inhibitors

Nitric oxide is of fundamental importance in many cellular interactions and has an important role in host defence and in many aspects of the immune response. Production by macrophages is important for protection from microbial infections. However, it also down-regulates Th1 cells and IFN-γ production, indirectly favouring Th2 proliferation. It has been suggested that the use of inhaled selective inhibitors of inducible NO synthetase (iNOS) inhibitors may reduce the dose of inhaled corticosteroids required for asthma control.

Further reading

Barnes PJ, Liew FY. Nitric oxide and asthmatic inflammation. *Immunology Today* 1995; 16: 128–30.

Barnes PJ. Cyclic nucleotides, phosphodiesterases and airway function. *Eur Resp J* 1995; 8: 457–62.

Cronstein B. Adhesion molecules in inflammation. Current research and new therapeutic targets. *Clin Immunother* 1994; 1: 323–26.

Leung DYM. Atopic dermatitis: the skin as a window into the pathogenesis of chronic allergic diseases. *J Allergy Clin Immunol* 1995; 96: 302–19.

Spector S. Leukotriene inhibitors and antagonists in asthma. *Ann Allergy Asthma Immunol* 1995; 75 :33–41.

Tanaka RD et al. Mast cell tryptase: a new target for therapeutic intervention in asthma. *Int Arch Allergy Immunol* 1995; 107: 408–409.

Bibliography

Allergy texts

Allergy Principles and Practice. Vols I & II. 4th ed. Elliot Middleton Jr, Charles E Reed, Elliot F Ellis, N Franklin Adkinson Jr, John W Yunginger, William W Busse (eds). Mosby, St Louis, 1993.
The classic authoritative multi-author, multi-volume textbook for reference purposes.

Samter's Immunologic Diseases. 5th ed. MM Frank, KF Austen, HN Claman, ER Unanue (eds). Little Brown, Boston, 1995.
A classic two-volume book, thoroughly updated by these eminent editors. Combines allergy with more clinical immunology than Middleton's 'Allergy Principles and Practice'. Highly recommended for reference.

Allergic Diseases: Diagnosis and Management. 4th ed. Roy Patterson (ed). JB Lippincott, Philadelphia, 1993.
Multi-author textbook of manageable proportions with a practical approach.

Allergy. Stephen T Holgate, Martin K Church (eds). Gower Medical Publishing, London, 1993.
An excellent British book, especially strong on underlying pathophysiology.

Atlas of Allergies. 2nd ed. Philip Fireman, Raymond G Slavin (eds). Mosby-Wolfe, Sydney, 1996.
Heavily illustrated. An excellent basic text.

Essential Allergy. An illustrated text for students and specialists. Niels Mygind. Blackwell Scientific Publications, Melbourne, 1996.
This book takes a novel and highly effective approach to the subject at an intermediate level. A second edition has just been published.

ABC of Asthma. 3rd ed. John Rees, John Price (eds). *BMJ,* via AMAS Medical Publications, Nedlands, 1995.

Immunology texts

There is a large selection, and only a few can be mentioned. Basic standard texts include:

Essential Immunology. 8th ed. Ivan M Roitt. Blackwell, Melbourne, 1994.

Cellular and Molecular Immunology. 2nd ed. Abul K Abbas, Andrew H Lichtman, Jordan S Pober. WB Saunders, Sydney, 1994.

Medical Immunology for Students. JHL Playfair, PM Lydyard. Churchill Livingstone, Edinburgh, 1995.

Basic and Clinical Immunology. 8th ed. DP Stites, AI Terr, TG Parslow. Appleton & Lange, Norwalk, Connecticut, 1994.

Slightly more advanced text but in the same illustrated format as Roitt's original book.

Immunology. Ivan M Roitt, J Brostoff, D Male. 4th ed. Times Mirror International, London, 1996.

Immunobiology. 2nd ed. CA Janeway, P Travers. Churchill Livingstone, Edinburgh, 1996.

Clinically oriented immunology texts are as follows:

Clinical Aspects of Immunology. 5th ed. Peter J Lachman, Sir D Keith Peters, Fred S Rosen, Mark J Walport (eds). Blackwell Scientific Publications, Melbourne, 1993.
Multi-author and multi-volume immunology text which is clinically orientated.
Essentials of Clinical Immunology. 3rd ed. H Chapel and M Haeney. Blackwell Scientific Publications, Melbourne, 1993.

Other books

Friendly Food. The complete guide to avoiding allergies, additives and problem chemicals. AR Swain, VL Soutter, RH Loblay. Allergy Clinic, Royal Prince Alfred Hospital. Murdoch Books, Sydney, 1991.
An illustrated book describing recipes and approaches to designing diets, of value for patients and professionals alike.

Dr Mike Smith's Postbag: Allergies. Written with Sharron Kerr. Kyle Cathie Ltd, 7/8 Hatherley St, London, 1994.
An excellent little book for patients.

Journals with frequent review articles in allergy

Modern Medicine of Australia
Very accessible and often has good review articles on allergy, mainly by Australian authors.

Medical journals, e.g. *New England Journal of Medicine; Journal of Allergy and Clinical Immunology; Annals of Allergy, Asthma and Immunology; Allergy; Clinical experimental Allergy; Allergy and Clinical Immunology News International.*

Immunology and Allergy Clinics of North America
An excellent annual publication of review articles on a wide variety of topics in allergy. Published by WB Saunders, Harcourt Brace Jovanovich, Philadelphia.

Appendices

1. Elimination diet for investigation of possible food intolerance or allergy

Explanation and objectives

As far as is practicable this diet aims to exclude:

(a) natural and added chemicals likely to be responsible for food intolerance such as salicylates, amines, sulphites, benzoates, preservatives and colouring agents such as tartrazine, azo and other dyes; and

(b) foods to which allergic reactions commonly occur.

The diet is intended to be followed for a period of two weeks. Over the course of this period improvement will gradually occur in the symptoms and the need for antihistamines will gradually subside. One of the indications that the diet has been effective is if these agents are no longer necessary.

At the end of this period if there has been no response in symptoms, the diet must be abandoned and a normal diet resumed. If there has been improvement, the investigation can proceed further by taking food chemicals disguised in capsules, or by adding single items of food back to the diet one by one every 48 hours and observing any reactions.

A diary should be kept of foods and drinks taken each day, and of symptoms. This should be presented to the doctor or dietician at each visit. Fruit and vegetables should be peeled thickly.

	Foods allowed	**Foods not allowed**
Beverages	Coffee—ground beans, for filter, drip or percolated	Instant and decaffeinated coffee, tea Herbal teas, cereal coffees Milo, Ovaltine, similar drinks
	Water Unflavoured mineral water, soda water Pear juice Whisky, gin, vodka	Flavoured mineral water, soft drinks Other fruit juices, cordials Wine, beer, cider, other spirits
Grains, bread and cereals	Rice cakes, rice flour bread Rice bubbles Tapioca, sago, arrowroot	All other breads, crumpets, muffins etc Muesli, other cereals Snack foods, e.g. crisps, corn chips, cheese snacks

—continued

	Foods allowed	**Foods not allowed**
Meat, fish, poultry	Lamb, veal, chicken (lean, no skin)	Beef, pork Corned, pickled meat Offal, including kidney, liver Sausages, processed meat, tinned meat, meat paste, pies Fish, other seafood.
	Eggs (if not allergic)	
Vegetables	Rice White cabbage Potatoes (old, brushed) Celery Lettuce Asparagus Shallots	Red cabbage Red Pontiacs, new potatoes Commercial potato crisps Cucumbers, capsicum Zucchinis Tomatoes Onions Peas, beans, lentils
Fruit	Pears (peeled) Golden delicious apples Bananas Paw-paw Pomegranate	Stone fruit, e.g. peaches, plums, apricots, nectarines Granny Smith apples Berries, e.g. strawberries, raspberries, blackberries, cherries Citrus, e.g. oranges, mandarins Kiwi fruit, gooseberries, mangoes Pineapple Imitation fruit flavours, e.g. cordials Dried fruit
Fats and oils	Margarine: Becel, Sundew (no milk products) Oil: sunflower, safflower, cold-pressed	Butter Other margarines Olive and other oils
Jams, spreads, flavourings	Golden syrup Maple syrup Pear and rhubarb jams Sugar Salt Malt vinegar Natural vanilla Parsley Garlic	Honey Low calorie jams Jams from other fruits Vegemite, Marmite, Promite Artificial sweeteners Wine and other vinegars Worcester, soy and other sauces Herbs and spices

	Foods allowed	**Foods not allowed**
Personal items/ medications	Paracetamol	Aspirin, NSAIDs, medicinal syrups and solutions, vitamins, other over-the-counter preparations
	Toothpaste: salt and soda Soul Pattison's unflavoured	

2. Some food additive numbers

Azo dyes and colouring agents

102	Tartrazine
110	Sunset yellow
127	Erythrosine
133	Brilliant blue FCF

Preservatives and additives

210–213	Benzoic acid and benzoates
220–224	Sulphur dioxide, sulphites, metabisulphites
249–252	Nitrites and nitrates
280–283	Proprionic acid and proprionates

Antioxidants

| 320 | Butylated hydroxyanisole (BHA) |
| 321 | Butylated hydroxytoluene (BHT) |

Flavouring agents

| 621 | Monosodium glutamate |

Adapted from: Approved food additive numbers. Published by National Health & Medical Research Council, available from dieticians at local hospitals, pharmacists, and Community Health Centres.

See also Hanssen M with Marsden Jill. *Additive Code Breaker.* Revised for Australia by The Commonwealth Department of Health. Melbourne: Lothian Publishing Company Pty Ltd, 1986.

3. Content of some clinically important chemicals in foods

Levels	Low	High
Naturally occurring chemicals		
Salicylates	Milk, soy milk, coffee	Tea, cereal coffees, cordials
	Gin, whisky, vodka Pear juice	Beer, wine, cider, cocoa, chocolate, tomato and fruit juices
	Beef, chicken, lamb, rabbit, veal	Smallgoods, pies, tinned tuna smoked meats and fish, offal
	Eggs, plain dairy foods, cottage cheese, cheddar cheeses	
	Peeled 'old' potatoes, white cabbage, lettuce, celery, brussels sprouts, shallots, chokoes	Red and new potatoes, cucumbers, zucchinis, capsicum, mushrooms, sprouts, onions, tomatoes, eggplant, dried peas, beans, lentils, radishes
	Rice	Bamboo shoots
	Vanilla, garlic, parsley	Other herbs and spices
	Golden syrup	Honey
	Malt vinegar	
	Flavoured toothpastes	
Amines	Fresh meats, white fish	Preserved smoked meats, offal, smallgoods
		Fish with coloured flesh or preserved fish, canned tuna
		Bananas, grapes, citrus, pineapple, plums, tomatoes, avocados, dates
		Chocolate, cocoa, colas
		Tasty cheeses, cheese flavours
		Sauces, stock cubes,
		Yeast and meat extracts, e.g. Vegemite

—*continued*

Levels   **Low**   **High**

Food additives
(Check containers for labels; see approved additive numbers)

Sulphites and   Fresh foods   Drinks, especially orange juices,
Metabisulphite   other fruit juices, commercial
(220–224)   fruit salads, wines, beers,
                                                   some spirits

                                               Stock and flavouring cubes and
                                                   packets, tomato preparations

                                               Commercial dressings

                                               Pickles, chutneys, mustards

                                               Cider and wine vinegars

                                               Dried fruits, including products
                                                   which contain them, e.g.
                                                   breads, cakes

                                               Low calorie jams, lemon butter,
                                                   marzipan

                                               Processed meats and cheeses

                                               Cake, biscuit and pastry mixes

                                               Hot potato chips, crisps

Monosodium glutamate (621)   Savoury snacks and frozen
(Also occurs naturally)   convenience foods

                                               Savoury/flavoured mustards,
                                                   sauces, e.g. Worcester,
                                                   barbeque, pickles, chutneys,
                                                   commercial stocks,
                                                   flavouring, tomato, tomato
                                                   paste

                                               Dehydrated foods, processed
                                                   meats, cheese spreads

                                               Some restaurant foods.

4. Antibiotic desensitisation protocols

Penicillin

The mechanism is probably antigen-specific mast cell desensitisation. Once desensitisation has been achieved dosing must be continued without a break. This is a dangerous procedure with a risk of serious anaphylaxis developing and is indicated only if penicillin is life-saving and there is no substitute. The patient must be under constant medical supervision with resuscitative measures in place. It should be undertaken only in a hospital setting. Mild reactions require the dose to be repeated, while more severe reactions may require return to a lower dose or cessation of the protocol.

Time*	Concentration mg/ml	Volume ml	Dose mg (subcut)	Cumulative dose mg
0	0.1	0.10	0.01	0.01
1	0.1	0.20	0.02	0.03
2	0.1	0.40	0.04	0.07
3	0.1	0.80	0.08	0.15
4	1.0	0.15	0.15	0.30
5	1.0	0.30	0.30	0.60
6	1.0	0.60	0.60	1.2
7	10	0.10	1	2.2
8	10	0.20	2	4.2
9	10	0.40	4	8.2
10	10	0.80	8	16.2
11	100	0.15	15	31.2
12	100	0.30	30	61.2
13	100	0.60	60	121.2
14	1,000	0.10	100	221.2
15	1,000	0.20	200	421.2
16	1,000	0.40	400	821.2
17	1,000	0.50	500	1321.2

Observe patient for 30 minutes. If no adverse reactions, proceed to intravenous

| 18 | 1,000 | IV | 0.5 g | 1821.2 |
| 19 | 1,000 | IV | 1.5 g | 3321.2 |

Continue with intravenous penicillin if no reaction.

* Interval between administrations 15 minutes.

Adapted from Sullivan TJ. *Current Therapy in Allergy, Immunology and Rheumatology.* Lichtenstein LM, Fauci AS (eds). London: The CV Mosby Co, 1985.

Sulphonamides (cotrimoxazole)

This is a dangerous procedure with the risk of inducing severe reactions. Its only indication is in patients with HIV infection and other rare instances in whom cotrimoxazole therapy is life-saving for treatment of *Pneumocystis carinii* infection. Patients with HIV infection have a higher risk of developing adverse reactions to cotrimoxazole and other drugs than the rest of the population. The challenges are given orally at 3-hourly intervals.The paediatric suspension is used and diluted appropriately. Highly diluted solutions should be made fresh each day.

Day	Time	Concentration mcg/ml	Volume ml	Dose mcg	Cumulative dose mcg
1	0	100	0.1	10	10
	1	100	0.2	20	30
	2	100	0.3	30	60
	3	100	0.4	40	100
	4	100	0.6	60	160
	5	100	0.8	80	240
	6	100	1.0	100	340
	7	100	2.0	200	540
2	0	100	3.0	300	840
	1	100	5.0	500	1,340
	2	100	7.5	750	2,090
	3	100	10	1,000	3,090
	4	100	20	2,000	5,090
		mg/ml	**ml**	**mg**	**mg**
	5	10	0.4	4	9.09
	6	10	0.8	8	17.09
3	0	10	1.5	15	32.09
	1	10	3.0	30	62.09
	2	10	5.0	50	112.09
	3	10	10	100	212.09
	4	10	20	200	412.09
		DS(double strength tablet)			
		Half DS tablet		400	812.09
		One DS tablet		800	1,612.09

4   One DS tablet (800 mg) four times a day

5   Two DS tablets (1,600 mg) three to four times daily depending on weight, continued for duration of treatment.

(This schedule is in operation at Concord Repatriation General Hospital, Sydney).

5. Useful addresses and resources

Hayfever and Allergy Information Service. The Service has published a series of simple brochures explaining various allergic conditions for the lay person. Available from many pharmacists, supplied to doctors for their waiting rooms, and available from the Hayfever and Allergy Information Service, PO Box 946, North Sydney NSW 2060.

Medic Alert. A non-profit organisation supplying personal emergency medical information systems. Australia Medic Alert Foundation, 216 Greenhill Road, Eastwood SA 5063.

Allersearch Asthma and Allergy Aids. Supply protective products including mattress and pillow coverings, and aids for allergy. Allersearch, 28 Martha Street, Granville NSW 2142.

Advice and many of these products available from many pharmacies which display their sign.

Bayer Australia Ltd. NSW. 2073. Suppliers of Acarosan miticidal preparations for carpets and furnishings, and desensitisation vaccines (Allpyral and Albay) Bayer Australia Ltd, Pharmaceutical Business Group, PO Box 903, Pymble, NSW 2073.

The *Asthma Foundation* in each State is an excellent resource.

Index

Page numbers in italics refer to illustrations or tables.

A

ABPA. See Aspergillosis
Acacia. See Wattle
ACE inhibitors
  and angioedema 127, 168
  and cough *86*
Acetyl salicylic acid. See Aspirin
Adenosine monophosphate, cyclic
      (cAMP) *215*
Adenyl cyclase 214, *215*
Adenosine triphosphate (ATP) *215*
ADHD 153, 193
Adhesion molecules. See Cell adhesion
      molecules
Adjuvants
  diesel particles 205
  alum 60
  latex 205
Adrenaline 44
  in anaphylaxis 141
  in asthma 101
Adrenocorticosteroids. See
      Corticosteroids
Air-conditioners
  in pollen avoidance 21
Air pollution. See Pollution
Air quality 91, 230
Airways
  bronchial, in children 92
Allergens
  avoidance 20
  definition 208, 223
  nomenclature *224*
  properties 223, 227
Allergic alveolitis. See extrinsic allergic
      alveolitis
Allergic facies 67, *68*
Allergic rhinitis. See also Rhinitis
  adverse reactions to foods 151
  prevalence 203, *204*
Allergic shiners *68*
Allergy
  biology 219, *221*
  definition 1, 3, 208

genetics 220
  prevention. See Prevention
  to the 20th Century (total allergy
      syndrome) 196
Alternaria 13, *224*, 232
Alum 60
Alveolitis. See Extrinsic allergic
      alveolitis
Amines 244
Aminophylline 101
Ampicillin, reactions to 172
Amoxycillin, reactions to 172
Anaphylaxis 3, 138
  causes 139, *140*
  emergency management *141*
  exercise induced 141
  idiopathic 141
  pathology 144
Anaesthesia and anaphylaxis 141
Androgens
  in hereditary angioedema 132
Angiotensin converting enzyme
      inhibitor. See ACE inhibitors
Angioedema 125
  causes 127
  due to ACE inhibitors 168
  investigation 129
Animal danders 176, *177*
Ant bites 157, 163
Antibiotics
  allergic reactions to 172
  in eczema 118
  in sinusitis 84
Antibodies
  blocking 54
  homocytotropic. See reagin
  IgE. See Immunoglobulin E
  IgG4. See Immunoglobulin G4
Anticholinergics
  antihistamines 30, 32, 36
  in asthma 101
  in rhinitis 74
Antidepressants
  antihistamine properties 38
  cardiotoxicity 38

N

NANC pathways 106
NARES 18, *66*, 69
Nasal cytology 18
Nasobronchial reflex 106
Nebulisers 25
Nedocromil sodium 26, 101
Nervous system
  autonomic
    in control of bronchial airways 106,
      107
    in control of nasal airways 77
    non-adrenergic non-cholinergic
      (NANC) 106
Neuropeptides in asthma 106
Neutrophils in allergic inflammation
    212
  in nasal secretions 72
Nickel 176, 223
Nitric oxide/NO 105, *206*, 219, *219*, 237
Nitric oxide synthetase inhibitors 237
Nonsteroidal antiinflammatory agents
    (NSAIDs) 90
Nose
  foreign bodies 70
  functional anatomy *76*
  functions 75
  neurovascular supply *77*
  polyps 82

O

Oatmeal preparations in eczema 116
Old man's drip 71
Olive tree pollen *224*, 232
Oral allergy syndrome 152
Otitis media 84
Oxygen therapy in asthma *100*

P

PAF. See Platelet activating factor
Parabens, reactions to 173
Parasite infection 4, 128, 129
Parasympathetic nervous system
  in bronchial airways 106
  in nose 77
Parietaria judaica 206, 231
Particulate matter 230
Patch testing 116
Paterson's curse 206, 229
Peak expiratory flow rate (PEFR) 11, 93

Peanut allergy 155
Penicillin
  allergy 171
    prevalence 205
  desensitisation 171, 246
Periactin. See cyproheptadine
Phadiatop[R] 16
Phosphodiesterase inhibitors 236
Photosensitivity 168
Pigeon breeder's lung 109
Plantain 232
Plasma cells 209
Platelet activating factor 101, 135
Platinum salts *177*
Plicatic acid 176, *177*
Pollen 227, 228, *229*
  anemophilous 229
  allergens
    classification *224*
  avoidance 60
  counts 231
  dispersal 229, 231
  entomophilous 229
  grass. See grass pollen
  sampling 228
  tree 229
Pollution
  effects on allergy 205
  effects on asthma 205
  Types I and II 205, 206
Polypectomy 83
Polyps, nasal 67, 82
  associated with asthma and aspirin
    hypersensitivity 82
  management 83
Postnasal drip 82, 85
Precipitins
  in extrinsic allergic alveolitis 109
Prednisolone, prednisone *41*
Pregnancy
  antihistamines in *37*
  diet in preventing allergic disease 58
  immunotherapy in 46
Prevention of allergy
  in infancy 58, *59*
  in adults 60
Priming effect of pollen exposure 227
Privet 231, 232
Profilin *224*, 225
Prostaglandins
  in asthma 105
  in pathogenesis of allergy 135, *216*
Prostaglandin D2 105
Provocation testing
  in adverse reactions to foods 154

X

X-rays. See radiology

Y

Yeast in Candida hypersensitivity
syndrome 197